THE SCAL METHOD:

(SAY CHEESE AND LIFT)

YOUR GUIDE FOR TOTAL BEING FITNESS

Evan Johnson

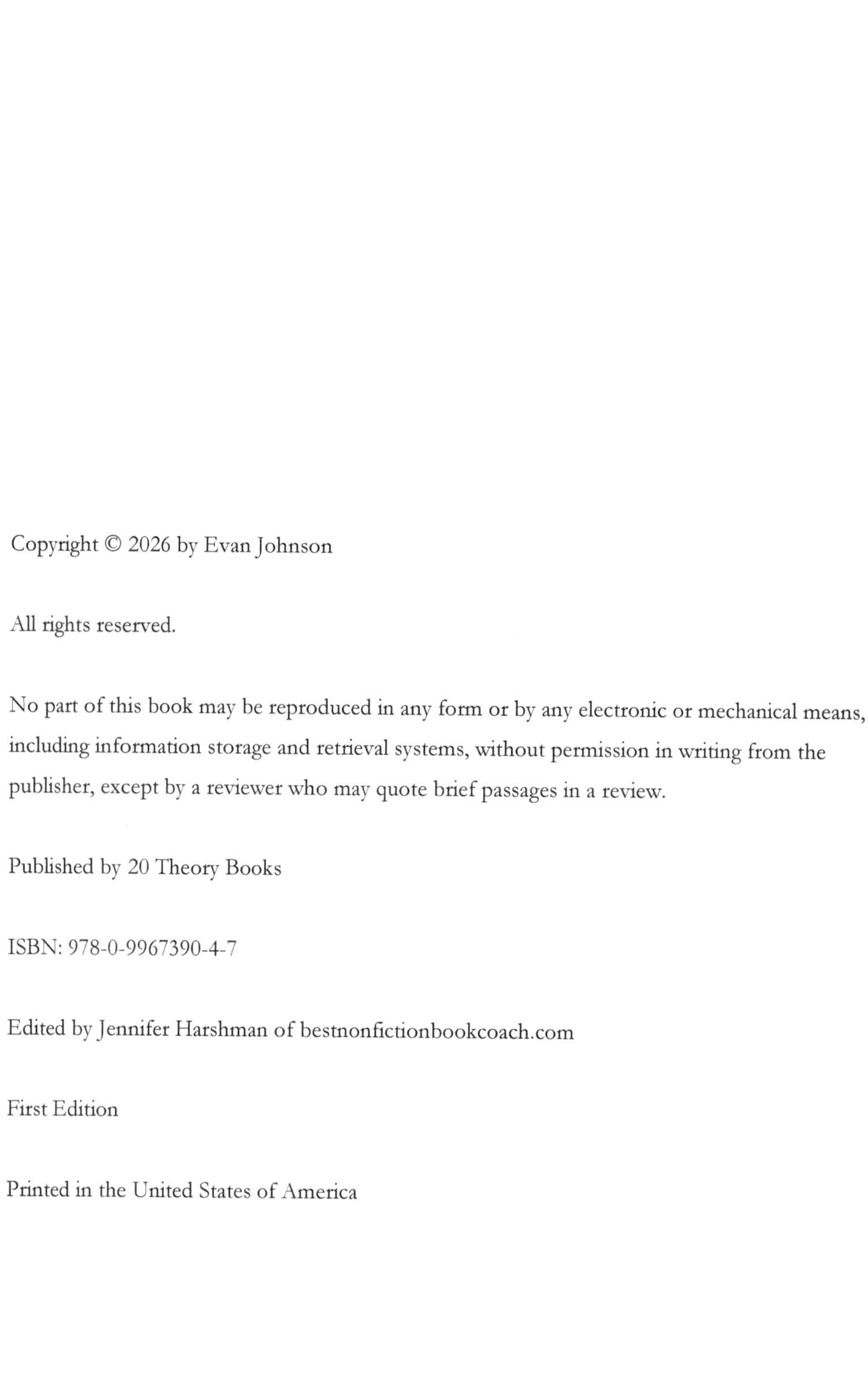

Published by 20 Theory Books

ISBN: 978-0-9967390-4-7

Edited by Jennifer Harshman of bestnonfictionbookcoach.com

First Edition

Printed in the United States of America

For Dad

CONTENTS

FOREWORD

As a pastor and missionary in ministries that involve trauma and other calamities that detour and derail people's lives, this body of work by Evan Johnson has been a jewel for building and healing the three components of spirit, soul, and body. The S.C.A.L. Method incorporates the step-by-step stages that help in fulfilling this verse: "A spirit of a man sustains him in sickness, but as for a broken spirit who can bear it?" (Prov. 18:14 Amp)

In the scholastic system of psychology, we are often made to believe that spiritual or religious beliefs are of little value to the mental stability and physical development of human life. One is considered philosophical, while the other scientific. However, the truth is that God created man in such a fashion that spirit, soul, and body are never independent of each other. To neglect one aspect is to impair the other. Many therapists have recognized this fact over the last 20 years or more and have included spiritual components in their healing and restorative strategies. Evan has embodied this knowledge in his approach to holistic healing. As a follower of Christ and one who has fought for over 30 years with Chronic Rheumatoid Arthritis, which causes severe joint pain and mental stress, the S.C.A.L. Method addresses that which many physicians and chemical treatments seem to miss—and believe me, I have been subject to many chemical treatments. I have found strength in these pages that have inspired me to fulfill God's command known as the Shema: "To love the Lord your God with all your heart, all your soul, and with all your strength" (Deut. 6:4).

Rev. Franklin C. Gilliam III

INTRODUCTION

For more than a decade, I've helped people achieve all kinds of health and fitness goals. Within a few years, I noticed a very curious pattern.

The clients who actually achieved their health goals—the ones who lost the weight, built the strength, and stuck with it long-term—didn't just follow the program I laid out for them. They made it more than a fitness thing.

Most of them were already happy. Most of them had someone pouring into them along the way, whether that was a mentor, a spouse, a community, or me. The ones who succeeded weren't just training their bodies. They were training something deeper . . . something greater.

At that point, I realized this wasn't a fitness thing at all, at least not in a traditional sense. There was this whole aspect of the human being that I wasn't coaching on.

So I started digging. I studied how the body works. I absorbed the studies on hormones, nervous systems, sleep patterns, inflammation, and more.

Then I dug into how that affects the mind—cognition, emotion regulation, decision-making. The more I learned, the clearer it became: you can't separate the body from the mind, the heart from the soul. They're one integrated system. Train one arena, and the others respond. Neglect one, and the others suffer.

Eureka! I cracked the code!

But in my personal life, I hit a wall.

Depression came for me like a storm I didn't see coming.

I kept training clients. But for myself? Workouts were stagnant. Thoughts were suffocating. I was angry at something and nothing at the same time. My prayers felt hollow, as if I were shouting into a void. My wife noticed the shift. My sons saw something but didn't know enough to comprehend what was going on.

I was helping others move forward while I was stuck in place, drowning in a darkness I couldn't name.

That's when The SCAL Method was born.

It wasn't born in a moment of triumph but one of desperation. I needed a way out of that suffocating fog, and nothing I'd been taught—not the fitness protocols, not the therapy sessions, not even the spiritual disciplines I'd practiced for years—was enough on its own. So I stopped treating them as separate. I started working all four arenas simultaneously: heart, mind, body, and soul. Not sequentially. Not one at a time. All at once.

Gradual Change

Little by little, the darkness lifted. My workouts came back to life. My thoughts cleared. My prayers stopped feeling like I was putting on a show and started feeling like a real connection. I wasn't fixed overnight, but I was moving again.

And my clients, whether they knew it or not, reaped the benefits. They became more resilient. They reached greater heights because they had someone pouring into them who was finally whole enough to give.

That's what this book is: the framework that brought me back to life, now tested and refined with hundreds of others.

Too many Christians live fragmented lives—praying for their souls while neglecting their bodies, sharpening their minds without reining in their hearts, serving faithfully while burning out silently.

We treat discipleship and stewardship as if they only apply to the "spiritual" parts of life, as if the body doesn't matter, as if emotions are optional, as if the mind can coast on autopilot.

Jesus commanded otherwise. He lived out a different reality.

WHOM THIS BOOK IS FOR

This book is for the person who senses the gap between what they profess and how they actually live (which, if we are being honest, we have to say is most of us). It's for those who know the right answers but still struggle with the daily discipline of loving God with their whole being.

You might be one of these people:

- A health-conscious person is burned out by optimization culture and looking for something that is sustainable. You're tired of performance metrics, biohacking rabbit holes, and self-improvement treadmills that promise transformation but deliver exhaustion.

- A believer prays faithfully but can't shake chronic anxiety. Their mind knows truth but their heart won't steady.

- A Christian has neglected physical health for years, saying, "The body doesn't matter," only to realize it does, and it's limiting their capacity to serve.

- The parent or spouse has unexamined emotions that are corroding relationships, leaving that parent or spouse reactive, defensive, and exhausted.

- The leader finds that their mental clarity has dulled, their discernment feels clouded, and their thinking has become lazy or reactive instead of sharp and wise.

- A gym goer is interested in integrated wellness, not just fitness, not just therapy, not just spirituality but a framework that takes all dimensions of human flourishing seriously.

If any or all of these describe you, this book is for you. Not because it has all the answers but because it gives you a biblical framework and practical tools to steward the whole person God made you to be.

WHAT WE MEAN BY "FITNESS"

When most people see the word *fitness*, they think of gyms. Reps and sets. Six-pack abs. Running times. Body composition. That's fair. I started as a personal trainer, so for years, that's what fitness meant to me too.

But I've come to learn that definition is too small.

The word *fitness* comes from the idea of being suitable, adapted, prepared. In biology, an organism is "fit" when it can survive and thrive in its environment. In machinery, parts are "fit" when they function as designed under stress. In Scripture, believers are called to be "fit for the Master's use" (2 Timothy 2:21), prepared and equipped for good works.

Fitness, properly understood, is about readiness. It is about having capacity. This alone gives you the ability to meet what life demands of you without breaking.

That's why this book is about Total Being Fitness; not because I'm diluting the term, but because I hope to restore it. Physical fitness was never supposed to stand alone. It was always pointing to something larger. Your body is one system among many.

Think about physical fitness for a moment. You can't build a strong body by only training one system. You need cardiovascular endurance, muscular strength, skeletal integrity, flexibility, and recovery. If you miss one, the whole system tends to suffer. A strong heart can't compensate for weak joints. Powerful legs don't fix poor lung capacity. "Boulder shoulders" cannot cover for trash recovery. I think you get my point.

The same principle applies to your entire being. You're not just a body. You're a heart that feels, a mind that thinks, a soul that worships. These arenas don't operate independently. They're intricately and meticulously woven together.

That's the theory. Of course, I had to learn this the hard way.

NOTE FOR NONCHRISTIANS

There are *many* Bible verses in this book. That's because this book is mainly for Christians and those accepting of the Christian worldview. If you're reading this and you don't identify as Christian, you can still get substantial value from the content.

The practical tools (emotional regulation, critical thinking, physical discipline, contemplative practice) are backed by mainstream science and apply universally. You don't need to share my faith to benefit from the framework. If you respect ancient wisdom traditions, are curious about integrated wellness, or are simply tired of one-dimensional approaches to human flourishing, you'll find practical strategies here that work regardless of belief.

Treat the Scripture as you would any wisdom literature—of course I would argue that it is way more than that. Still, test it against your experience, take what serves you, and adapt the rest to your own worldview. The body still keeps score. The heart still needs training. The mind still requires sharpening. And the deepest part of our being still anchors everything.

WHY THIS BOOK NOW

We live in a strange moment. The wellness industry is booming—meditation apps, fitness influencers, self-optimization gurus—all promising wholeness through technique. Meanwhile, the church often responds by retreating into the "spiritual," as if caring for the body or training the mind is a secular distraction.

Both miss the mark.

The wellness industry, in large part, ignores the soul. It offers strategies without the anchor of worship, techniques without the tether of truth. It trains the body and mind but leaves the deepest part of you—the part where God meets you—untouched and unformed.

The church, too often, ignores the body. We tend to spiritualize everything, treating physical discipline as optional or even suspect, as if holiness has nothing to do with how you sleep, what you eat, or whether you move. We reduce discipleship to Bible study and prayer while ignoring the physical dimension of being human.

Oftentimes, the emotional and intellectual dimensions are used to the extreme. Either they are neglected, or the opposite:

how one feels and what one thinks replace spiritual cognition (the soul's capacity to recognize, interpret, and integrate things revealed to the human spirit) altogether.

We are more anxious, more exhausted, and more disconnected than ever. We need an integrated approach—one rooted in Scripture, not self-help; one that takes the body seriously without idolizing it; one that honors the soul without neglecting or worshiping the mind and heart.

That's what The SCAL Method offers: whole-person discipleship for a fragmented age.

THE FOUNDATION

Jesus answered:

"Love the Lord your God with all your heart and with all your soul and with all your mind and with all your strength. The second is this: 'Love your neighbor as yourself.' There is no commandment greater than these" *(Mark 12:30–31).*

This is it. The blueprint. The Great Commandment. Heart, soul, mind, strength—four arenas of human existence, named by Christ himself. Not suggestions. Not helpful tips. Commands. And beneath the command is a design: you are meant to love God with your whole being, and that whole being has structure.

The SCAL Method is built on this foundation. It doesn't add to Scripture or improve on it. It simply takes Christ's command and maps practical discipleship onto the four arenas he identified. Sound heart. Sound mind. Strong body. Strong soul. Each one matters. Each one requires stewardship. Each one shapes the others.

This is not a self-help system. It is not optimization for its own sake. It is discipleship that takes seriously the dimensions of being human. You cannot love God with your mind if your mind is clouded by anxiety. You cannot serve him with your body if your body is wrecked by neglect. You cannot guard your heart if you have never trained it. You cannot nourish your soul if you treat it as an afterthought.

The SCAL Method takes holistic wellness seriously because Scripture does. What you do with your heart, mind, body, and soul matters. It either strengthens your capacity to love God and neighbor, or it weakens it.

The Four Arenas

A Sound Heart

Your heart is not a nebulous concept. It is the control center for your emotions.

"A sound heart is life to the body, but envy is rottenness to the bones" (Proverbs 14:30).

A sound heart shows up time and time again in the form of disciplined emotional regulation—the ability to feel without being ruled by feeling.

When your heart is trained, your words are steady. Your decision-making sharpens. Your presence stabilizes. An untrained heart corrodes everything to your very core.

A Sound Mind

Your mind is the seat of wisdom, discernment, and clarity.

"For God hath not given us the spirit of fear but of power, and of love, and of a sound mind" (2 Timothy 1:7).

A sound mind is not just intelligent; it is wise. It thinks critically, weighs evidence, questions assumptions, and seeks truth. It refuses confusion, laziness, and reactivity. A trained mind strengthens the heart, guides the body, and anchors the soul.

A Strong Body

Your body is a temple, and temples require maintenance.

"Your bodies are temples of the Holy Spirit . . . honor God with your bodies" (1 Corinthians 6:19–20).

A strong body is not vanity. It is proper stewardship. Physical discipline builds mental resilience, stabilizes emotions, and creates capacity for service. Neglect your body, and you limit your ability to serve. Train it, and you extend your runway.

A Strong Soul

Your soul is the deepest part of you, the place where God meets you.

"He restores my soul" (Psalm 23:3).

A strong soul is nourished through prayer, Scripture, worship, and community. It is the anchor that steadies the heart, informs the mind, and energizes the body. Neglect your soul, and everything else becomes brittle. Nourish it, and resilience flows outward.

ARENA INTERCONNECTION

The four arenas are not separate compartments but one complete system. What happens in one arena ripples into the other arenas, always. Seriously. Always.

Heart → Mind

Unchecked emotions cloud judgment. Anxiety narrows focus. Resentment distorts perception. When the heart is chaotic, the mind cannot think clearly. But when the heart is trained—when emotions are named, accepted, analyzed, expressed, and reframed—the mind gains clarity. Emotional regulation is cognitive training.

Mind → Heart

The mind shapes the heart through reframing. When you challenge distorted thoughts, you disrupt destructive emotional patterns. When you rehearse truth, you steady the heart. Romans 12:2 tells us to renew our minds. The mind is the lever that moves the heart.

Body → Heart & Mind

Physical discipline stabilizes emotions and sharpens thinking. Movement reduces cortisol, improves sleep, and interrupts anxiety spirals. Strength training builds mental grit. Endurance work teaches you to sit with discomfort. A trained body creates the conditions for a steady heart and a clear mind.

Soul → Everything

The soul is the foundation. Prayer steadies the heart. Scripture sharpens the mind. Worship aligns affections. Community provides accountability. When the soul is nourished, resilience flows into every other arena. When the soul is neglected, everything else becomes fragile.

This is not sequential. It is simultaneous. You don't master one arena before starting another. You work all four at once, knowing that progress in one strengthens the others.

FRAMEWORK AS DISCIPLESHIP

Discipleship involves both inner transformation and outward practice. This doesn't just apply to the soul but every aspect of our existence.

Jesus didn't just save souls; he healed bodies, challenged minds, and commanded hearts. The gospel is holistic. Discipleship must be as well.

The SCAL Method is a framework to be more Christlike across all four arenas. It refuses the false divide between "spiritual" and "physical," between "emotional" and "intellectual." It takes seriously the biblical truth that you are made whole, and God calls you to love Him with your whole self.

Training the heart is discipleship. Emotional regulation is not self-help; it is sanctification. Guarding your heart (Proverbs 4:23) means training it to respond to truth instead of reactivity. It means learning to name envy before it corrodes, to accept grief without suppressing it, to reframe distortions before they take root.

Training the mind is discipleship. Critical thinking, intellectual humility, and the pursuit of truth are acts of worship. The mind is trained through study, questioning, testing assumptions, and wrestling with complexity. Wisdom directs it toward truth and love. Together, they form the capacity for discernment that honors God and serves others.

Training the body is discipleship. Your body is a temple (1 Corinthians 6:19–20), and caring for it is an act of worship. Physical discipline—strength training, endurance work, rest, nutrition—is stewardship. It is not vanity. It is preparing yourself to serve longer, think clearer, and love more steadily.

Training the soul is discipleship. Prayer, Scripture, worship, and community are not optional add-ons. They are the foundation. Psalm 23:3 says God restores the soul. Restoration requires a cadence of practices that keep you anchored. You cannot skip the soul and expect the rest to hold.

The SCAL Method is not a program. It is a way of life that takes the Great Commandment seriously. Love God with all your heart, soul, mind, and strength. This framework isn't mere philosophy; it gives you concrete practices that train each arena.

COMMON OBJECTIONS

Before we go further, let's address some objections. Over the years, I've heard many. You may already be thinking some version of these common objections:

"I don't have time."

This isn't about adding more. It's about stewarding what you already have. You already have a heart. Train it. You already have a mind. Sharpen it. You already have a body. Care for it. You already have a soul. Nourish it.

The SCAL Method doesn't demand hours; it demands intentionality. Start with small moves. Take three minutes, or do ten pushups, read one verse, name one emotion. Time is not the issue. Discipline is.

"I've tried programs before."

This is not a program. Programs promise results in 12 weeks. They offer techniques detached from true discipleship and stewardship. The SCAL Method is a framework for life, rooted in the Great Commandment. It's not about finishing; it's about faithfulness. You don't "complete" loving God with your whole being. You show up daily, year after year, training the four arenas that Scripture names.

"Isn't this just self-help?"

No. Self-help is technique without a deeper guiding purpose, optimization without worship. It trains the body and mind but leaves the soul untouched.

The SCAL Method starts with the soul and works outward. Prayer anchors the heart. Scripture sharpens the mind. Physical discipline extends your capacity to serve. This is not self-improvement; it is whole-person alignment under the lordship of Christ.

"This sounds overwhelming."

It's not. I'm not calling you to become masterful in each arena by tomorrow. I'm asking you to start with one micro move in each arena. That's it. Then tomorrow, do it again. Progress is not measured in perfection but in steady rehearsal. In other words, I'm looking for consistency of effort.

HOW TO USE THIS BOOK

This book is structured around the four arenas, each chapter walking you through the biblical foundation, the science, and the practice. Here's what lies ahead:

Chapter 1: A Sound Heart

You'll discover why your unexamined emotions are wrecking your relationships, clouding your judgment, and corroding your body. You'll learn the five-step process for training your heart: Name. Accept. Analyze. Express. Reframe. You'll gain tools for emotional intelligence (EI) and see how a sound heart produces and improves life in every arena.

Chapter 2: A Sound Mind

You'll learn to think critically, weigh evidence, question assumptions, and distinguish truth from noise. You'll see how wisdom is cultivated, not inherited, and how sharpening the mind strengthens discernment, steadies the heart, and anchors the soul. You'll receive strategies for defeating mental laziness and protecting your mind from distraction.

Chapter 3: A Strong Body

You'll see why neglecting your body limits what you can do and shortens the time you'll have to be of service in this world. You'll gain practical strategies for strength, endurance, rest, and nutrition—not as vanity but as stewardship. You'll discover how physical discipline stabilizes emotions, sharpens thinking, and extends your capacity to love and serve.

Chapter 4: A Strong Soul

You'll learn how to nourish the deepest part of you through prayer, Scripture, worship, and community. You'll see how a strong soul anchors everything else and provides the resilience needed to train the heart, sharpen the mind, and strengthen the body. You'll receive tools for defending spiritual practices in a distracted world.

Chapter 5: Endurance and Strategic Discomfort

You'll discover why comfort kills growth and how strategic discomfort builds capacity across all four arenas. You'll learn to embrace endurance, not as punishment, but as a refining tool. You'll gain additional tools for pressing into difficulty and emerging stronger.

Chapter 6: Relationships

You'll see how training the four arenas transforms your relationships. A sound heart steadies your words. A sound mind sharpens your discernment. A strong body extends your patience. A strong soul grounds your love. You'll learn how to love others well by first discipling yourself well.

Each chapter includes these:

- **Biblical foundation**—Scripture anchors every principle.

- **Scientific validation**—Modern research confirms ancient wisdom.

- **Practical tools**—You can implement concrete strategies today.
- **Practice prompts**—Short exercises build the habit. Next to each practice, you'll find this symbol:.

Along with sources at the end, there's a comprehensive verse list, detailing every Bible verse used in the book (a big help for studies).

Remember, knowledge is not the goal. Transformation is.

You can read this book and change nothing. Or you can make one micro move today and begin a process that will help you reshape your life.

STEWARDSHIP =/= PERFECTION

This is not a performance-based system. You will not master all four arenas. You will not arrive. We are not looking for perfection.

Stewardship means working with what you have been given. God gave you a heart, mind, body, and soul. You are responsible for what you do with these gifts.

The parable of the talents (Matthew 25:14–30) makes this clear. The servants who stewarded well were commended. The one who buried his talent (skills, opportunities, resources, time) was condemned—not for failing to multiply it tenfold but for doing nothing. Stewardship is not about perfection or even results; it is about faithfulness.

Start where you are. Choose one small move to make in each arena. Show up tomorrow. Do it again. The fruit will come, but it comes through faithfulness.

THE PRACTICE PROMPTS

Every chapter includes practice prompts. These aren't suggestions. They're assignments. And they work best when you track them.

Get a notebook. Doesn't matter if it's fancy or cheap. Physical or digital. Just something you'll actually use. This is your SCAL journal.

When you hit a practice prompt, write your responses in the journal. Date them. Be specific. Don't write, "I need to work on my heart." Write, "I felt resentment toward my boss Tuesday afternoon, when he interrupted my presentation. Analyzed it: felt disrespected and overlooked. Reframed it: he's under pressure from leadership and wasn't targeting me personally."

The journal does three things:

It forces clarity. Thinking about something and writing it down are different. Writing forces you to get specific. Specificity is where change happens.

It tracks patterns. After a month, you can flip back and see which emotions keep surfacing, which decisions keep tripping you up, which physical habits keep slipping. Patterns reveal blind spots.

It creates accountability. When you write down your commitment on Monday and review it on Friday, you can't lie to yourself about whether you followed through. The journal keeps you honest.

Some prompts ask you to share your response with an accountability partner. Do it. Text them the actual words from your journal. Don't summarize. Send the screenshot. Accountability without specifics is just check-ins that go nowhere.

Start your journal today. Date the first page. Write, "Beginning The SCAL Method." Then use the practice prompt at the end of this Introduction as your first entry.

PRACTICE PROMPT

Write down one micro move for each arena:
- Heart: Name one emotion you felt today.
- Mind: Read one verse, and ask one question about it.
- Body: Do ten pushups or take a ten-minute walk.
- Soul: Pray for three minutes.

Success Criteria

☐ You tracked your progress and reviewed your notes.

Troubleshooting

If naming emotions feels impossible, start with physical sensations instead (tightness, heat, heaviness). The words will come. If you're stuck, use an emotion wheel to expand your vocabulary.

THE ROAD AHEAD

The stakes are high. Your heart shapes your relationships, and your mind shapes your discernment. Your body shapes your capacity to serve, and your soul shapes everything. What you do with these four arenas matters; not just for you but for everyone God has called you to love and serve.

So begin. Not tomorrow. Today. Choose one tiny thing to do in each arena. Take one step. Show up.

Love the Lord your God with all your heart, soul, mind, and strength. There's the command. Our blueprint.

Alright, let's get busy!

CHAPTER ONE
A SOUND HEART

"A sound heart is life to the body, but envy is rottenness to the bones" (Proverbs 14:30).

It was 5:27 AM when my phone sounded off. Immediately, I knew something was wrong because it wasn't the sound of my alarm. But my phone wouldn't sound off if it wasn't one of the key four people: My Mom, Dad, brother, or wife. I picked up.

It was my brother, and he sounded frantic.

"I tried. They're here trying resuscitate him."

"What?" I could barely understand what he said.

"It's Dad."

I'll spare you all of the details, but my father died that day, suddenly. That changed my life forever. And it all happened not long before I finally pulled together this book. But why is this opening the chapter on a sound heart? One simple word is the answer: grief.

You see, this is only the second real death that I had to deal with, the first being my grandmother. And when my grandmother passed away from cancer, I pushed on. I thought if I threw myself into my work, I would be okay. I believed I was doing good work, after all. But I found myself sad and sick more often. I felt my purpose slipping away from me. My grandmother's death is one of the main catalysts to that dark unnamed depression I spoke of in the opening.

As I was studying, praying, researching, building The SCAL Method, I came across this thing called grief bypass. It hit me in the face harder than Anthony Joshua hit Jake Paul. I'd never sat with the loss of my grandmother. I'd never grieved. I'd never lamented over my grandmother's death. And it kept coming up in so many places again and again.

So, I determined in my mind not to do that. My wife and children couldn't live through that twice. They didn't and still don't deserve that. Even then, it took some more prompting from some key individuals in my life to put that determination into action.

I took a trip to the middle of nowhere, Pennsylvania, to a cabin on a creek. No phone or TV. No work or programs. Just my Bible and my prayer journal (and some food and clothes, of course). Oh! And I also brought with me a book by a man named Leonard Ravenhill: *When Revival Tarries*. I spent my days and nights praying, crying, and hiking. I grieved. And I prayed. And I listened. And I read. But one thing I did not do is try to breeze by it. I didn't try to reframe this crappy situation as something else because I didn't fully understand what I felt. That was only my second time grieving.

It felt like the whole first day, I cried, the wails coming from deep within my soul.

And then I recognized what I was feeling in its entirety. Yes, I absolutely felt grief. But I also felt regret. He and I wanted the same things: to take care of those closest to us, to walk in the purpose that God has set for us, but we both went about those things in very different ways. And for that, we butted heads a lot. Quite frankly, I never took the chance to tell him that I understood him, that I respected him, and that I loved him no matter what. Then there was frustration because there were too many people around who were judging him based on things they could never understand. It all came into focus.

But eventually, I found I was at peace. I was finally able to let my buddy go. Then, I was able to reframe. And that led me to being able to live a fuller life without running up on those landmines of suppressed emotion. My father's passing taught me a bunch more, but maybe I'll save that for another book.

My point here is that I was able to regulate, not suppress or ignore, the mix of emotions I felt after his passing.

So, a sound heart is not a slogan. It's not a feeling, per se. It's disciplined emotional regulation—the ability to feel without being ruled by feeling.

Let me be plain: having **a sound heart is having the proper regulation of your emotions.** Period. That's the definition. Remember it.

Think of it as a rhythm instead of chaos. Numbness silences the music; steadiness keeps the beat. A sound heart is relaxed and resilient, and it changes how your body carries itself in the world. This matters because if you want the rest of life—relationships, service, ministry, leadership—to hold together, you start here. Another way to look at it is as the control tower where decisions are cleared for takeoff, where speech and action receive their orders.

Proverbs 14:30 presses the point:

"A sound heart is life to the body, but envy is rottenness

to the bones" (Proverbs 14:30).

The Hebrew word for "sound" (marpeh/rafeh) leans into healing and restoration. This isn't just calmness; it's repair. The proverb ties soul condition to body condition. Your emotions don't stay hidden. They move into your cells. That's the gospel's hard edge: neglect the heart, and the body pays the price.

Here's what that looks like in real life: You carry resentment toward your boss for three months. You think you're hiding it well. Meanwhile, your blood pressure climbs, your shoulders stay tense, and you snap at your kids over nothing. The body keeps score. Always. An unchecked heart corrodes everything downstream: your sleep, your digestion, your relationships, your witness.

And Proverbs 4:23 adds urgency:

"Above all else, guard your heart, for everything you

do flows from it" (Proverbs 4:23).

Guarding is not avoidance. It is stewardship. It means regulating what enters and what rules. Guarding your heart is the act of naming envy before it corrodes, refusing bitterness before it takes root, and keeping the interior life aligned with truth. Proper emotional regulation is the practical way you guard the heart so that what flows out—words, choices, relationships—carries life instead of decay.

CONNECTION TO THE METHOD

A sound heart doesn't work in isolation. It's the foundation for everything else:

- **Sound Mind:** Unchecked emotions cloud judgment. Train the heart, and the mind thinks clearer.
- **Strong Body:** Chronic stress from emotional chaos wrecks sleep, immunity, and recovery. A regulated heart stabilizes the body.
- **Strong Soul:** Spiritual practices require emotional honesty. You can't pray with integrity if you're lying to yourself about what you're feeling.

A sound heart produces life. An unsound heart breeds corrosion. What rules the heart ripples outward into speech, decisions, and presence.

PRACTICE PROMPT

- ❖ Write a sentence that defines "sound heart" in your words.

- ❖ List one area of life (a relationship, your work, or your ministry) where emotional steadiness would change outcomes.

Success Criteria

☐ You wrote your definition.
☐ You identified the specific area where emotional steadiness would change outcomes.
☐ You read it aloud with conviction.

☐ Within twenty-four hours, you texted it to someone who knows you well.

Troubleshooting

If you can't bring yourself to text it, ask why. That resistance reveals how much you're performing versus how honest you're willing to be regarding this.

If the person you texted responded with something generic, you picked the wrong person. Find someone who will actually call you on your patterns, not just affirm you.

EXEGESIS

Proverbs 14:30 speaks with precision. Let's break it down. This text doesn't fall into the abstract category. It directly names the emotion of envy, forcing us to see soundness as an emotional condition. The imagery is physical—life coursing through the body versus decay eating away at the bones. Scripture ties the unseen interior to the visible exterior, showing that what rules the heart eventually shows up in the flesh.

The Hebrew word for "sound" (*marpeh/rafeh*) carries the sense of cure, peace, and restoration. It is the language of healing, not passivity. In contrast, "rottenness" is a vivid picture of corrosion. This proverb is a sort of diagnostic on your system. It tells us that unmanaged emotions are not harmless—they are destructive forces that seep into health, relationships, and witness.

Why Precision Matters: Envy vs. Jealousy

Clarity matters. Envy and jealousy are often blurred together, but they are distinct. Confusing them is like calling a fracture a bruise—you'll treat it wrong and make it worse.

- **Envy** resents what another possesses.
- **Jealousy** protects what is valued and perceived as threatened.

Confusing the two collapses moral categories. Envy corrodes because it breeds comparison and bitterness. Jealousy, though dangerous if unchecked, can be a protective instinct toward covenant or calling. God himself is described as jealous (Exodus 34:14). God is not envious. He protects what is rightly His.

Sarah sees her colleague get promoted. If Sarah feels **envy**, she resents her colleague's success and lets bitterness grow. If Sarah feels **jealousy**, she's protecting what she values—her own calling and contribution—and the emotion signals, "I need to clarify my role here or have a conversation with my boss."

One corrodes. One can be constructive if stewarded. But only if you name it accurately.

Precision in naming emotions is part of guarding the heart. Mislabeling them is like misdiagnosing an illness—the wrong treatment follows. Guarding the heart means guarding categories. If envy is disguised as jealousy, corrosion is excused. If jealousy is mislabeled as envy, protective instincts are condemned.

Scripture demands accuracy. The heart cannot be trained if the emotions ruling it are misnamed. This is where EI becomes critical—the skill of perceiving and naming emotions with precision. More on that later, because the ability to discern and manage feelings is the engine that makes the whole thing work.

How This Strengthens the Mind

This precision work—distinguishing envy from jealousy, naming emotions accurately—is cognitive training. You're building the same mental muscle you need for critical thinking, for discerning truth from error, for making wise decisions under pressure.

PRACTICE PROMPT

- ❖ Write down two emotions you've confused in the past (for example, envy versus jealousy or anger versus grief).

- ❖ Define each in one sentence.

- ❖ Then note how mislabeling them changed your response.

Success Criteria

☐ You wrote down two emotions you've confused.
☐ You defined each in one sentence.
☐ You noted how mislabeling changed your response
☐ You tracked every time the emotion showed up this week.

☐ You reviewed your notes at week's end to identify patterns.

Troubleshooting

If you can't identify emotions you've confused, you're either emotionally precise (rare) or emotionally unaware (common). Ask someone who knows you, "Do I ever say I'm angry when I'm actually hurt?" They'll know.

If tracking feels impossible, you're not pausing long enough. The emotion appears, you react, it's gone. Slow down the sequence.

PHYSICAL CONSEQUENCE

Unchecked emotions are not neutral. They are corrosive forces that eat away at daily functioning. Scripture warns that envy rots the bones, but the principle extends further: resentment inflames, anxiety disrupts sleep, grief unsettles the body. What begins in the heart does not stay hidden. It moves into the bloodstream, the nervous system, the rhythms of rest and work.

Untrained emotions are like cancer: they spread quietly until they weaken every system they touch.

The Physical Reality

Resentment is a slow poison. It raises blood pressure, stiffens posture, and narrows perception. You think you're just "not a fan" of someone.

Meanwhile, your jaw is clenched, your shoulders are up around your ears, and you're scanning every conversation for evidence that they're out to get you.

Anxiety is a thief of rest. It hijacks sleep cycles, floods the body with cortisol, and leaves the mind racing when it should be recovering. You lie awake at 2 AM replaying a conversation that hasn't happened yet. The body is exhausted, but the mind won't shut down.

Grief, when suppressed, does not disappear; it lodges in the body, weakening immunity and draining energy.

You tell yourself, "I'm fine. I've moved on." But you're getting sick more often, your energy is flat, and you can't figure out why.

These are just some of the physical consequences that show

up in fatigue, inflammation, and relational breakdown.

Science Catching Up

Modern science confirms what Scripture told us thousands of years ago. Chronic anger strains the cardiovascular system. Anxiety disorders alter hormone balance and disrupt digestion. Suppressed grief leaves the body vulnerable to illness.

The heart is not a metaphorical container; it is the command center that sets the body's pace. When emotions are left untrained, the body pays the bill.

Studies show that chronic emotional dysregulation correlates with the following:

- Higher cortisol levels (stress hormone)
- Increased inflammation markers
- Weakened immune response and wound healing
- Disrupted sleep architecture
- Higher cardiovascular disease risk

The research is clear: your emotional state shapes your physical state. Always.

THE HEART–BODY–MIND LOOP

This is where Heart, Body, and Mind form a loop. Unchecked anxiety (Heart) disrupts sleep and raises cortisol (Body), which clouds judgment and triggers catastrophic thinking (Mind), which amplifies the anxiety. The loop accelerates.

Training the heart breaks the cycle. A sound heart stabilizes the body, which steadies the mind, which reinforces emotional resilience. The loop reverses direction. This is why stewardship of the interior life is not optional.

THE STAKES

Training emotions is not about slogans or quick fixes. It is about longevity—the ability to serve, to lead, to witness, and to love without burning out or breaking down. A sound heart is life to the body because it sustains clarity, resilience, and strength. An unsound heart corrodes health, fractures relationships, and clouds the person's judgment.

Guarding the heart is guarding your future. It's also guarding your capacity to love others well. It's hard to be patient with your kids when your nervous system is fired. Serving with joy is difficult when resentment is eating you from the inside.

PRACTICE PROMPT

❖ Take one emotion you've struggled with recently (anger, envy, grief, or anxiety). Write down how it showed up in your body: tension, sleeplessness, fatigue, or pain. Be specific. Where exactly did you feel it? When?

❖ Then note how mislabeling them changed your response. fused in the past (for example, envy versus jealousy or anger versus grief).

❖ Write one way that training that emotion could change your health and your relationships.

Success Criteria

☐ You identified a recent emotion and wrote down how it showed up physically with specific details (where in your body, when it happened).

☐ You noted one way training that emotion could change your health and relationships. Share this with your doctor at your next appointment.

Troubleshooting

If you can't connect emotions to physical symptoms, you're disconnected from your body. Start by noticing: tight chest, clenched jaw, tense shoulders, shallow breathing.

If you're avoiding the doctor conversation because it feels awkward, that awkwardness is exactly why you need to do it. Doctors know this connection exists; bringing it up shows self-awareness, not weakness.

GROUNDWORK AND SEQUENCE

Emotions are not enemies. They are signals. Left untrained, they become noise; trained, they become clear messages. The heart's soundness depends on whether emotions are stewarded with discipline or allowed to run unchecked.

Scripture commands us to guard the heart. Modern psychology confirms that emotional regulation is the foundation of resilience. Training emotions is not about suppression—it is about stewardship, guiding the emotions into alignment with truth and purpose.

Here's the framework. Five steps. Memorize them. Practice them daily. They work.

Name → Accept → Analyze → Express → Reframe

Let me show you what this looks like with a real example, then we'll break down each step.

Real-World Example: Sarah

Sarah is a worship leader. She arrives at church Sunday morning to find the tech team didn't set up her mic correctly—again. She feels a surge of anger, snaps at the sound guy, and then feels guilty during worship. She spends the rest of the day replaying it, beating herself up. Here's how the five-step sequence would have changed that morning:

Name: "I feel angry. Actually, I feel disrespected."

Accept: "I'm feeling disrespected right now. That's real. I'm not going to spiritualize it away or pretend I'm fine."

Analyze: "The trigger was the mic setup. But why disrespect? I believe that if they cared about worship, they'd get it right. And maybe I believe that if they cared about me, they'd pay attention."

Express: Before snapping, Sarah takes 30 seconds. She texts her accountability partner: "Tech messed up again. I'm about to lose it. Pray for me." She prays honestly: "God, I'm angry. I feel disrespected. Help me respond with patience."

Reframe: "One mistake is not a verdict on their commitment or my worth. They're volunteers who showed up early on a Sunday. I can address the pattern this week without attacking them now. My response in the next two minutes matters more than the mic."

Sarah still addresses the issue but with measured speech instead of a snap. She serves well during worship. She brings it up calmly with the team lead on Tuesday.

That's the sequence in action. Now let's break it down.

1. Name.

The first step is recognition. You cannot train what you don't name. Proverbs 4:23 calls us to guard the heart, and guarding begins with clarity. Naming emotions is like identifying intruders at the gate. Anger, envy, grief, anxiety—each must be called by its proper name.

Why This Matters

Vague language keeps you stuck. "I feel bad" is useless. "I feel rejected" or "I feel resentful" is actionable. Mislabeling them leads to confusion and mismanagement. If you think you're stressed when you're actually afraid, you'll try to solve the wrong problem.

What To Do

When an emotion hits, pause for five seconds. Ask: "What am I actually feeling?"

Not "fine," "stressed," or "whatever." Name it with precision:

- Anger? At what specifically?
- Envy? Of whom, for what?
- Fear? Of what outcome?
- Grief? Over which loss?
- Shame? About what action or identity?

Naming is the act of honesty, the refusal to hide behind vague language when corrosion is already at work.

How This Strengthens the Mind

Precision in naming emotions trains precision in all thinking. This is cognitive discipline disguised as emotional work. Every time you accurately name an emotion, you're building the same mental muscle you need for clear thinking, wise decision-making, and resisting manipulation.

2. Accept.

Naming without acceptance leads to denial. Acceptance is not indulgence; it is acknowledgment.

To accept an emotion is to admit its presence without shame. Psalm 42 shows the psalmist speaking directly to his own soul:

"Why are you cast down, O my soul?" (Psalm 42).

That is acceptance—facing the reality of sorrow.

Why This Matters

Repression doesn't kill emotions; it drives them deeper into the body, where they manifest as fatigue, tension, or illness. You can't heal what you won't acknowledge. Acceptance prevents that corrosion.

What we resist persists. What we accept, we can work with.

What To Do

After naming the emotion, say it out loud if you're alone, or write it down if you're not: "I am feeling angry right now."

Not "I shouldn't feel this way." Not "This is stupid." Not "Good Christians don't feel like this." Just: "I am feeling ___."

That single sentence stops the spiral of shame that makes emotions toxic. Shame says, "You're bad for feeling this." Acceptance says, "You're human for feeling this."

How This Strengthens the Soul

Acceptance before God is the posture of honest prayer. You can't confess what you won't admit. The Psalms are full of raw, honest emotion: anger at God, despair, complaint. David doesn't spiritualize; he names and accepts. This is the groundwork for spiritual integrity.

If you can't be honest with God about what you're feeling, your prayer life will boil down to nothing but performance, a far cry from intimacy.

3. Analyze.

Acceptance opens the door to analysis. Analysis asks questions like the following:

- Where did this emotion come from?
- What triggered it?
- What belief sustains it?

Proverbs 14:30 ties envy to bodily decay, showing that emotions have roots and consequences. Analysis is the act of tracing those roots. Was envy triggered by comparison? Was anger fueled by unmet expectations?

Why This Matters

Most emotional reactions are not about the trigger; **they're about the belief underneath.** Sarah's anger wasn't really about the mic. It was about her belief that mistakes equal disrespect.

You don't get angry at every mic failure. You get angry when the failure means something to you. Analysis reveals the meaning you've assigned.

PRACTICE PROMPT

- ❖ Ask three questions:

  - **What triggered this emotion?** (The mic setup. The email. The conversation. Be specific.)
  - **What belief made that trigger hurt?** (Mistakes mean they don't care. Criticism means I'm failing. Delay means rejection.)
  - **Is that belief actually true?** (Not necessarily. They're volunteers. Mistakes happen. Other explanations exist.)

- ❖ Write down your answers. **The act of writing forces precision.**

Analysis is not overthinking; it is diagnosis. Just as a physician examines symptoms to find the cause, the steward of the heart examines emotions to uncover their source.

This is the Question Ladder from Sound Mind training applied to emotions. You're building analytical muscle every time you trace roots. You're learning to distinguish data from interpretation, fact from story. This skill transfers to every area of thinking.

4. Express.

Emotions must be released, or they stagnate. Expression is the act of channeling emotions into healthy outlets.

Scripture models this in the Psalms, where lament, praise, and petition give voice to the full range of human feeling. Science confirms that journaling, prayer, and verbal processing reduce stress and improve clarity.

Why This Matters

Unexpressed emotions don't disappear. They leak out sideways — in passive-aggression, in physical symptoms, in relational distance, in Sunday afternoon blowups over minor things.

Expression is controlled release. It's choosing the outlet instead of letting the emotion choose for you.

Venting without structure just rehearses the pain. Structured expression moves it out and lets you work with it.

PRACTICE PROMPT

Choose your outlet before the emotion hits.

- ❖ **Journaling:** Write it raw. Three pages. Don't edit. Get it out. No one will read it. This is for you and God.

- ❖ **Prayer:** Pray the emotion honestly. "God, I am angry. Here's why . . ." The Psalms give you permission. God already knows. Tell him anyway.

- ❖ **Trusted conversation:** Call your accountability partner. Say the thing out loud: "I need to process something. Can I talk for five minutes without you fixing it?" Then say what you're feeling.

- ❖ **Physical release:** If the emotion is highly charged,

move first. Walk, lift, run. Let the body burn off some of the cortisol. Then come back to another form of expression.

Expression is not venting without restraint; it is structured release. It is the difference between shouting in anger and praying in anger. One corrodes, the other heals.

How This Strengthens the Body

Releasing emotions through healthy outlets lowers cortisol, reduces muscle tension, and improves sleep. The body needs you to move emotion out, not store it. When you express emotions structurally, you literally change your biochemistry. Cortisol drops. Parasympathetic nervous system engages. The body can finally rest.

5. Reframe

The final step is reframing — aligning emotions with truth.

Romans 12:2 calls us to be transformed by the renewing of the mind. Reframing is that renewal applied to emotions. It asks, "How can this feeling be redirected toward growth, service, or wisdom?"

Why This Matters

The story you tell about a moment determines how that moment rules you. Change the story, and you change the emotional charge.

Reframing is not denial. You're not pretending nothing happened. You're changing the meaning you assign so the event no longer controls you.

Two people experience the same rejection. One tells a story of unworthiness. One tells a story of redirection. The second person recovers faster and grows more.

What To Do

After expressing the emotion, write a one-sentence reframe that does the following:

- Acknowledges reality (Don't deny what happened.)

- Challenges the automatic interpretation (Question the belief.)
- Redirects toward action (What can you do now?)

Examples:

Hurt

- Old story: "They ignored me. I don't matter to anyone."
- Reframe: "One person's oversight is not a verdict on my worth. I'll ask directly for what I need."

Rejection

- Old story: "They said no. I'm not good enough. I'll never succeed."
- Reframe: "One person's no is data, not destiny. I'll refine my approach and look for other doors."

Envy

- Old story: "They have what I want. Life is unfair. I'll never get ahead."
- Reframe: "Their gain highlights my desire. I'll use that desire to define a specific next step instead of stewing in bitterness."

Anxiety

- Old story: "I'm going to fail. Everyone will see I'm a fraud."
- Reframe: "This nervousness shows I care about doing well. I can use it to prepare thoroughly."

Anger

- Old story: "They violated a value I hold dear. I need to destroy them."
- Reframe: "This anger shows something important was violated. I can address it clearly without attacking."

Grief

- Old story: "This loss broke me. I'll never recover."
- Reframe: "This loss teaches me what matters. I can honor it by living more intentionally."

Reframing does not erase the emotion; it redeems it, turning corrosion into strength.

How This Strengthens the Soul

Reframing toward truth is the practical work of renewing the mind. This is sanctification—becoming more like Christ through the discipline of aligned thinking. When you reframe, you're asking: "What does Scripture say about this? What is actually true?" You're submitting your automatic thoughts to the authority of truth. That's discipleship.

WHY THIS SEQUENCE MATTERS

Without training, emotions rule the heart and corrode the body. With training, they become allies in service, leadership, and witness.

The **Name → Accept → Analyze → Express → Reframe** sequence is not a formula; it is a rhythm. It gives structure to the interior life, ensuring that emotions are neither suppressed nor indulged but stewarded. This rhythm produces resilience, clarity, and longevity. It is the practical way to guard the heart so that everything flowing from it carries life.

PRACTICE PROMPT

Choose one emotion you've experienced this week, and walk it through the full sequence, writing out each step in detail.

- ❖ **Name:** Write down the emotion with precision. Avoid vague words like "bad" or "upset." For example, instead of "I'm stressed," write, "I feel anxious about tomorrow's meeting." The goal is clarity: naming the intruder at the gate so you know what you're dealing with.

- ❖ **Accept:** Admit the emotion without shame or denial. Acceptance is acknowledgment not indulgence. For instance, "I feel anxious, and that's real." This step prevents repression, which only drives emotions deeper into the body.

❖ **Analyze:** Ask yourself where the emotion came from, what triggered it, and what belief sustains it. For example, "I feel anxious because I believe I might fail in front of others." Write down the trigger and the underlying belief. This is diagnosis: tracing the roots.

❖ **Express:** Channel the emotion into a healthy outlet such as prayer, journaling, or trusted conversation. For example, pray honestly about the anxiety or write it out in a journal. The goal is release: moving the emotion out of the body into words.

❖ **Reframe:** Align the emotion with truth. Ask how the feeling can be redirected toward growth or wisdom. For example, "My anxiety shows I care about doing well. I can reframe it as motivation to prepare." Reframing redeems the emotion, turning corrosion into strength.

❖ Write down each step in sequence. Notice how the emotion changes as you steward it.

Success Criteria

☐ You chose one specific emotion from this week.
☐ You wrote out each step of the sequence in detail (Name, Accept, Analyze, Express, Reframe) with concrete language.
☐ You spent twenty to thirty minutes on the exercise because you went deep, not surface-level.

Troubleshooting

If you rushed through this in five minutes, you skimmed the surface. Real emotional work takes time and feels uncomfortable.

If you couldn't identify the underlying belief in the Analyze step, you stopped too early. Keep asking, "Why?" until you hit the core belief.

If Reframe feels like you're lying to yourself, you're forcing positivity instead of aligning with truth. Truth isn't always positive, but it's always grounding.

REFRAMING DISCIPLINE

Reframing is the discipline of altering meaning to reduce emotional charge. It is not denial or wishful thinking; rather, it is the deliberate act of changing the story you tell about a moment so the moment stops ruling you.

At its core, reframing asks, **"What meaning am I assigning, and how true is that meaning?**

When the meaning shifts, the emotional intensity often follows.

The Two Core Reframe Types

Two high-value reframes anchor this practice: **positive reframing** and **evidence-based reappraisal**.

Positive reframing looks for upside, lesson, or gratitude in a hard situation—the "What did this teach me?" move. It doesn't deny the pain; it asks what good can be extracted.

Evidence-based reappraisal interrogates the story with data, testing negative interpretations against facts rather than feelings. It asks, "What evidence supports this story? What evidence contradicts it?"

Each has its place. Gratitude without reality testing can slip into denial. Data without gratitude can harden into cynicism. Used together, they balance one another, producing both truth and resilience.

Shaping the Big-Picture Layout

At the schema level, reframing interrupts automatic meaning. Schemas are the mental maps that supply instant interpretations when triggers hit. Left unchecked, they recycle old narratives:

"I'm worthless."

"I always fail."

"No one cares."

Reframing deliberately interrupts those scripts and offers new ones. Over time, this reshapes narrative patterns so that old triggers carry less charge. The long game is not just changing surface thoughts but rewriting the deeper maps that drive them.

Solid Science

The evidence is consistent. Systematic reviews confirm that

reframing and reappraisal support resilience, improve mood, and correlate with better mental-health outcomes when they are practiced reliably.

Neuroimaging studies show that reappraisal strategies recruit prefrontal control processes that modulate limbic reactivity, explaining why practiced reframes reduce felt intensity over time. This is not a trick; it is a skill that rewires response patterns.

The Micro-Protocol for Reframing

Here's the step-by-step process:

- **Name the event and your initial story in one sentence.** "My boss canceled our meeting, and that has to mean I'm being phased out."

- **Pause and ask for alternate meanings.** "What else could this mean? Could she be swamped? Could she have forgotten? Could this be about her and not me?"

- **Test the story with evidence.** Evidence supporting: She's canceled twice this month. Evidence contradicting: She praised my work last week. She's launching a new product line and everyone knows she's buried.

- **Create a truthful, one-line reframe that reduces charge and increases agency.** "One canceled meeting is not a verdict. She's in launch mode. If this becomes a pattern, I'll ask her about it directly."

- **Anchor the reframe in gospel truth or a corrective identity statement, paired with a pragmatic next step.** "My worth is not tied to her attention. I am loved by God and valued for who I am, not what I produce."

- **Decide on a next step:** "I'll send her a quick note saying I understand she's swamped and asking when we can reschedule."

Sample Reframes in Action

Let me give you fuller examples so you can see the before and after:

Example One: Hurt

My friend didn't text me back for three days.

Old story: She doesn't care about me. I'm always the one who cares more.

Evidence against: She responded within hours last month. She drove me to the airport when I needed help. She's dealing with a sick parent right now.

Reframe: One delayed response is not a verdict on our friendship. She's in crisis mode with her mom. I'll check in again and offer support instead of assuming rejection.

Gospel anchor: My worth isn't determined by response times. I am deeply loved by God. I can extend grace.

Next step: I'll text her: "Hey, no rush on replying. Just wanted you to know I'm praying for your mom. Let me know if you need anything."

Example Two: Rejection

I wasn't chosen for the job.

Old story: They didn't hire me. I'm not good enough. I'll never get the job I want.

Evidence against: They said they had 200 applicants. My resume got me to the final three. I've been hired for similar roles before.

Reframe: One company's no is data, not destiny. I made it to the final round, which means I'm competitive. I'll refine my interview approach and keep looking for the right fit.

Gospel anchor: God's plan for me is not thwarted by one hiring decision. He orders my steps. This no might be protecting me from a wrong fit.

Next step: I'll ask for feedback from the hiring manager. Then I'll apply to three more positions this week.

Example 3: Envy

Someone in my department received a promotion.

Old story: They got promoted. I've been here longer. Life is unfair. I'm stuck.

Evidence against: They led two major projects successfully. They've been networking intentionally. My performance reviews have been good but not exceptional.

Reframe: Their promotion highlights what I want. Instead of resenting them, I'll use this as clarity: I want more responsibility. I'll ask my manager what it would take for me to be considered next time.

Gospel anchor: God's gifts to others are not threats to me. There is enough blessing to go around. I can celebrate them and pursue my own calling.

Next step: I'll congratulate them genuinely. Then I'll schedule a meeting with my manager to discuss my career trajectory.

Reframing as a Discipline

Reframing is a discipline, not a one-time fix. Practiced consistently, it shifts the baseline of emotional life, turning corrosion into clarity and resilience. This is stewardship. You're not pretending pain doesn't exist. You're refusing to let pain write the final story.

How This Strengthens the Mind

Every reframe is a logic exercise. You're testing assumptions, weighing evidence, and drawing conclusions. This is critical thinking applied to emotions. The more you practice, the sharper your thinking becomes in every area.

How This Strengthens the Soul

Anchoring reframes in gospel truth roots emotional regulation in spiritual formation. You're not just managing feelings; you're aligning your inner life with the character of God. That's discipleship.

PRACTICE PROMPT

- ❖ Choose one recent sting or disappointment. Write down your initial story in one sentence.

- ❖ Pause and generate at least two alternate meanings.

❖ Test the story with evidence, listing facts that support and contradict the initial interpretation.

❖ Create one truthful reframe that reduces charge and increases agency.

❖ Anchor it in Scripture or a corrective identity statement, then write one pragmatic next step.

❖ Repeat this exercise daily for a week and note how your emotional charge shifts.

Success Criteria

☐ You identified one situation that typically triggers a strong emotion.
☐ You wrote out your standard reframe based on Scripture or another source of truth.
☐ You practiced saying it aloud three times daily for seven consecutive days.
☐ When the situation occurred, you actually used the reframe.

Troubleshooting

If you completed the exercise but the reframe didn't help, you chose a surface-level reframe instead of one that addresses your core belief. Go deeper. If you didn't practice daily, you're treating this like information instead of training. Repetition is required for rewiring.

If the situation triggered you and you forgot to use the reframe, your habit isn't strong enough yet. Add a cue: set a phone reminder, write it on a card you carry, or tell your accountability partner to text you the reframe daily.

COMMON REFRAMING PITFALLS

Reframing is a discipline, but like any discipline, it carries risks when misapplied. These pitfalls must be named clearly so the practice remains truthful, constructive, and aligned with both resilience and integrity.

Pitfall 1: Denial

Reframing must never collapse into false peace. If the new story erases reality, it is denial, not resilience.

Example

Your marriage is in crisis. Your spouse has said clearly they're unhappy. You reframe it as: "Everything's fine. We just need a vacation." That's denial. A truthful reframe would be: "We're in trouble. This is real. I need to face it honestly and get help."

Denial may feel soothing in the moment, but it corrodes trust, prevents genuine healing, and leaves the underlying issue untouched. True reframing acknowledges pain while redirecting meaning toward growth.

How to Avoid It

Test your reframe with one question: "Am I telling the truth, or am I protecting myself from the truth?" If you're not sure, ask someone who loves you enough to be honest.

Pitfall 2: Scapegoating

Reframing cannot be used to shift blame. Turning every negative event into someone else's fault is not stewardship; it is avoidance.

Example

You missed a deadline at work. You reframe it as: "My boss gave me too much. This is her fault for overloading me." Maybe she did overload you. But if you didn't communicate your limits, you own part of the story.

Scapegoating distorts responsibility, blocks growth, and damages relationships. Healthy reframing requires ownership of your part in the story, even when others contributed to the pain.

How to Avoid It

Ask, "What is my part here?" Even if someone else is 90% responsible, own your piece. This is important. The reframe must include your agency.

Pitfall 3: Grief Bypass

Reframing is not a substitute for grief work. When sorrow is acute, lament and processing are necessary. To reframe prematurely is to bypass grief, leaving wounds unhealed and compassion undeveloped.

Example

You lose a close friend to death. Someone tells you, "Just thank God for the time you had." That might be true eventually, but said too soon, it's grief bypass. First, you need to sit in the loss. First, you need to lament.

John 11:35 records the shortest verse in Scripture:

"Jesus wept" (John 11:35).

Even knowing Lazarus would be raised, Jesus wept. Grief is not a problem to be reframed away; it is a process to be honored.

True resilience requires facing loss honestly before reframing it into meaning.

How to Avoid It

When loss is fresh, give yourself permission to grieve first. Weeks or months later, you can ask, "What did this loss teach me? How can I honor it?" But don't skip the lament.

Pitfall 4: Acute Emotion Protocol

When emotions are raw and overwhelming, reframing should not be the first move. Safety, naming, and somatic regulation come first—grounding the body and stabilizing the heart.

Example

You just got terrible news. Your hands are shaking. Your mind is racing. Someone says, "Let's reframe this." No. First, breathe. First, feel your feet on the ground. First, name the emotion: "I'm terrified." First, let your body settle.

Breathing, movement, or supportive presence may be required before cognitive work is possible. Only once composure is regained can reframing be applied effectively.

How to Avoid It

If you can't take a full breath without shaking, you're not ready to reframe. Regulate the body first. Then return to cognitive work.

Example of a Pitfall Corrected

Situation

A pastor loses a long-time church member suddenly.

Grief Bypass (wrong)

He says, "God's timing is perfect. I'm just going to trust and move forward."

Three months later, he's irritable and distant from his family, and he can't figure out why. It's because he bypassed the grief.

Truthful Sequence (right)

- Weeks one and two: He grieves. He weeps. He prays lament psalms. He tells God he's devastated.

- Weeks three and four: He names the loss and what it means. He journals about the hole left behind.

- Weeks five and six: He begins to reframe: "This loss reminds me how fragile life is. I want to love my people more intentionally while I have them."

- Week twelve: He preaches on Psalm 23 with depth he didn't have before because he walked through the valley.

That's grief honored and not bypassed. That's reframing done right.

PRACTICE PROMPT

- ❖ Think of one time you tried to "spin" a painful moment. Write down the reframe you used. Then test it against the four pitfalls:

  - Did it deny reality? (Am I pretending it didn't happen?)

  - Did it scapegoat? (Am I blaming someone else to avoid my responsibility?)

  - Did it bypass grief? (Am I rushing to the lesson before sitting with the loss?)

  - Was it attempted too soon? (Was I still shaking when I

tried to reframe?)

- ❖ Revise the reframe so it is truthful, responsible, and timed appropriately.
- ❖ Notice how the corrected version feels different in your body and in your outlook.

Success Criteria

☐ You chose one recurring negative thought.
☐ You identified the distortion.
☐ You wrote the truth-based reframe.
☐ You used that reframe every time the thought appeared for five out of seven days.
☐ By day seven, you noticed the thought losing power or frequency.

Troubleshooting

If the thought still has the same power on day seven, you're not actually reframing when it shows up. You're thinking about reframing, which isn't the same thing. The moment the thought appears, stop, speak the reframe out loud if possible, and redirect. If you can't identify the distortion, you're not examining the thought closely enough. Are you indulging in all-or-nothing thinking? Catastrophizing? Personalization? It's there.

PRACTICE SCHEDULE

Reframing is not a one-time skill but a discipline that becomes effective only through repetition. To guard the heart and reshape schemas, it must be practiced consistently across contexts. A structured schedule ensures that reframing moves from occasional effort into habitual resilience.

Daily Practice (five minutes)

Set aside five minutes each day for reframe journaling. Choose one small sting or disappointment. Write down the initial story, list evidence for and against it, and create one truthful reframe.

This daily rhythm builds reflexive skill, training the mind to interrupt automatic narratives quickly. Five minutes. Every day. Non-negotiable.

Weekly Review (twenty to thirty minutes)

At the end of each week, identify three recurring triggers. Walk each through the micro-protocol: name, pause, test, reframe, anchor.

This weekly review highlights patterns and strengthens schema-level change, ensuring that repeated triggers lose their corrosive charge over time.

Example: You notice that every time your spouse is late, you spiral into "they don't respect my time." After three weeks of reframing, the trigger loses power. You start defaulting to saying, "They're running behind. I'll use these ten minutes to pray."

Monthly Narrative Work (sixty to ninety minutes)

Once a month, map the larger schemas that keep returning — the deep stories that shape your responses. Create corrective reframes for each, anchored in Scripture and identity statements.

This long-form work rewrites the underlying maps, not just surface thoughts, producing lasting transformation.

Examples:

- "I'm not enough."
- "People always leave."
- "If I'm not perfect, I'm worthless."

For each one, write:

- The pattern
- Evidence it's not universally true
- A gospel-rooted reframe
- One behavior change that reflects the new belief

Community Feedback (Monthly or as needed)

Invite trusted voices to review your reframes. External feedback prevents clever but false narratives and keeps the practice grounded in truth.

Reframing is most effective when practiced in community, where accountability and perspective sharpen discernment.

Example: You think your reframe sounds truthful. Your accountability partner says, "That sounds like you're letting yourself off the hook. Try again." That correction is gold.

Integration with Prayer (Daily)

After each reframe, hand it to God in prayer. Name the feeling, state the reframe, and ask for strength to live it out.

This integration turns cognitive discipline into spiritual formation, ensuring reframing is not mere self-management but part of guarding the heart.

Example prayer: "God, I felt rejected when they didn't include me. I've reframed it as this: their choice isn't a verdict on my worth. Help me believe that. Help me walk in the truth that I am loved by you. Give me the grace to respond with kindness, not bitterness. Amen."

PRACTICE PROMPT

- ❖ Design your own reframing schedule for the next month. Write these down:
    - Daily: When will you do five-minute reframe journaling? (Morning with coffee? Before bed?)
    - Weekly: What day/time will you do your twenty-minute review? (Sunday evening? Friday afternoon?)
    - Monthly: When will you do sixty to ninety minutes of narrative work? (First Saturday? Last Sunday?)
    - Accountability: With whom will you share reframes? When will you meet?

- ❖ Share your plan with a trusted friend or mentor for accountability.

- ❖ At the end of the month, reflect on how your emotional charge has shifted.

Success Criteria

☐ You read through all five pitfalls and identified which one describes you most accurately right now (not which one you *wish* was your problem).
☐ You wrote a specific recent example showing you in that pitfall.
☐ You implemented the correction within forty-eight hours.

Troubleshooting

If no pitfall resonates, you're either in rare emotional health, or you're blind to your patterns. Ask your spouse or close friend which pitfall they see in you. Their answer matters more than yours.

If you identified the pitfall but didn't correct within forty-eight hours, you're still living in it. Knowledge without action is another form of avoidance.

A LEVEL DEEPER

Emotional intelligence is the deeper engine behind a sound heart. It is a set of trainable skills that allow you to perceive, use, understand, and manage emotions with precision.

Unlike raw temperament, EI can be cultivated through deliberate practice, making it central to the discipline of guarding the heart.

What Emotional Intelligence Does

Emotional intelligence is the ability to do these things:

- **Perceive** emotions accurately in yourself and others.
- **Use** emotions to facilitate thinking and decision-making.
- **Understand** emotions—their causes, patterns, and likely outcomes.
- **Manage** emotions to achieve goals and maintain relationships.

This is not about being emotional or unemotional. It's about being skilled with emotions—reading them accurately, using them as data, and regulating them with discipline.

Why It Matters

The five-step sequence (Name → Accept → Analyze → Express → Reframe) depends entirely on EI. If you can't perceive emotions accurately, you can't name them. If you don't understand their patterns, you can't analyze them. If you can't manage them, you can't reframe them effectively.

Emotional intelligence is the engine. The sequence is the vehicle. Without the engine, the vehicle doesn't move.

COACHING FRAMEWORK

Developing EI requires structured training. Five pillars form the framework:

1. Vocabulary Expansion

Building a richer emotional lexicon allows you to name feelings with accuracy.

The Reason

Most people operate with a vocabulary of five to ten words for emotions: happy, sad, mad, scared, stressed. That's like trying to paint with five colors. Expanding your vocabulary gives you 50+ words: anxious, resentful, envious, disappointed, ashamed, content, grateful, tender, fierce, etc.

The Practice

Write down three new feeling words each week and use them in journaling. Instead of "I'm stressed," write, "I'm overwhelmed." Instead of "I'm sad," write, "I'm grieving."

Over time, precision grows. Precision enables regulation.

2. Early Detection

Learn to notice emotions at their onset rather than only after escalation.

The Reason

By the time you're yelling, you've missed ten earlier signals. The goal is to catch anger when it's irritation, anxiety when it's unease, and grief when it's a tightness in your chest.

The Practice
Do a body scan three times a day. Ask, "What am I feeling right now? Where is it in my body?" Notice sensations:

- Jaw clenched? (Anger brewing)
- Shoulders tight? (Stress accumulating)
- Chest heavy? (Sadness present)
- Stomach tight? (Anxiety rising)

The earlier you catch it, the easier it is to regulate.

3. Causal Mapping
Tracing emotions back to triggers and beliefs, identifying root causes instead of surface reactions.

The Reason

Most emotional reactions are not about the trigger; they're about the belief underneath. If you don't trace the root, you'll keep reacting to the same triggers over and over.

The Practice

Do some antecedent journaling: write down what happened immediately before an emotion arose. Do this for two weeks. Patterns will emerge.

Here is an example pattern: "Every time someone interrupts me, I feel disrespected. The trigger is interruption. The belief is: if they interrupt, they don't value me."

Once you see the pattern, you can test the belief.

4. Toolbox Practice
Rehearsing strategies such as reframing, breathwork, and constructive expression until they become reflexive.

The Reason

Under stress, you default to what you've practiced. If you've never rehearsed a reframe, you won't do it in the moment. If you've never practiced breathwork, you'll forget when panic hits.

Do breathwork: Practice four-seven-eight breathing daily (four seconds in, seven seconds holding, eight seconds out). Do it when you're calm so it's automatic when you're not.

- ❖ **Reframe:** Write five reframes this week, even if you're not emotional. Build the muscle.

- ❖ **Role play:** With a trusted partner, rehearse responses to common triggers. "What would you say if your boss canceled on you again?" Practice the calm response aloud.

Rehearsal builds reflexes.

5. Social Rehearsal

Practicing emotional regulation in community settings, where feedback sharpens discernment.

The Reason

Private practice is essential, but you don't know if your emotional regulation is working until you test it in relationships. Social rehearsal gives you real-time feedback.

PRACTICE PROMPT

- ❖ Ask a trusted friend, "Can we do a hard-conversation exercise? I want to practice staying calm when I'm challenged."

- ❖ Debrief after emotional moments: "How did I come across in that conversation? Was I defensive? Clear? Harsh?"

- ❖ Invite correction: "If you see me reacting emotionally instead of responding thoughtfully, would you call it out?"

Community keeps you honest.

INTEGRATING

Emotional intelligence is not isolated from other disciplines. It integrates directly with the following:

- **Breathwork:** Labeling emotions accurately will lower reactivity. Naming "I'm anxious" while breathing deeply calms the nervous system.

- **Cognitive reappraisal:** Understanding emotions helps you test the beliefs driving them.

- **Social correction:** Trusted friends help you see blind spots in how you perceive and express emotions.

Together, these practices form a comprehensive system for training the heart.

How This Strengthens the Mind

Every time you accurately perceive and name an emotion, you're building cognitive precision. You're learning to distinguish data from interpretation, signal from noise. That skill transfers to all thinking.

How This Strengthens the Body

Early detection prevents emotional escalation, which in turn prevents cortisol spikes, which protects sleep, immunity, and cardiovascular health. The body benefits directly from EI.

How This Strengthens the Soul

Emotional intelligence enables honest prayer. You can't confess what you can't perceive. You can't lament what you can't name. Emotional intelligence is the foundation for spiritual integrity.

PRACTICE PROMPT

Choose one recurring emotion you often mislabel. Then do the following practice.

- ❖ **Expand your vocabulary:** Find a more precise word for the emotion you are feeling. (Instead of "stressed," maybe "overwhelmed" or "anxious" or "scattered.")

- ❖ **Journal the antecedent:** What happened right before you started feeling that emotion? Write it down whenever it happens, for a week.

- ❖ **Question it three times:**
  - Why did that trigger hurt?
  - What made it hurt?
  - Where did that belief come from?

- ❖ **Rehearse a healthier response:** With a trusted partner, practice what you'll say/do next time that emotion arises.

- ❖ **Notice the shift:** See how accuracy and rehearsal change the way the emotion feels and flows.

Success Criteria

□ You chose one specific recurring emotion, named it precisely using a more accurate word than your default label, and wrote down what triggered it at least three times over the week.
□ You completed all three "why" questions in writing, traced the emotion to an underlying belief, and rehearsed a healthier response out loud with a trusted person — not just in your head.

Troubleshooting

If no pitfall resonates, you're either in rare emotional health or you're blind to your patterns. Ask your spouse or close friend which pitfall they see in you. Their answer matters more than yours. If you identified the pitfall but didn't correct within forty-eight hours, you're still living in it. Knowledge without action is another form of avoidance.

TOOLS AND INTEGRATION

Training the heart requires portable moves that can be deployed in real time, but those moves gain their deepest power when tied to prayer and Scripture. Tools without spiritual anchoring risk becoming mere self-management; spiritual practices without concrete tools risk remaining abstract.

Together, they form a complete system for guarding the heart.

Tool 1: Micro-Pause

It helps to take a short pause before reacting. You'll be more likely to respond appropriately rather than react reflexively.

What To Do

Inhale for four counts, exhale for six. Name the feeling in one word, then ask a clarifying question: "What story am I telling right now?"

This interrupts automatic reaction and creates space for choice.

When to Use It

When you feel the surge of emotion and you're about to speak or act. The pause is the difference between wisdom and regret.

How it Integrates

The micro-pause is a mini version of the full sequence. You're naming (perceiving), questioning (analyzing), and choosing (regulating)—all in ten seconds.

Tool 2: One-Sentence Reframe

Distorted thoughts gain power through repetition. A concise reframe disrupts the distortion and restores truth in real time.

What To Do

Craft a concise truth that reduces emotional charge. Here are some examples:

- "This setback is data, not destiny."
- "One person's no is not a verdict on my worth."
- "I can feel afraid and still act with courage."

The brevity forces clarity and makes the reframe portable in your daily life.

When To Use It

When you catch yourself spiraling into catastrophic thinking. Speak the one-sentence reframe out loud. Repeat it three times.

How it Integrates

This is Romans 12:2 in practice—renewing the mind with truth. The one-sentence reframe is your go-to weapon against lies.

Tool 3: 90-Second Reset

Emotions surge through the body before they settle in the mind. This reset lowers intensity so you can respond instead of react.

What To Do

Step away from the trigger for ninety seconds. Breathe, recall a gospel anchor, and let the body settle.

Research shows that the physiological lifespan of an emotion is about 90 seconds if you don't feed it with more thoughts. After 90 seconds, the intensity naturally decreases if you let it.

This short reset lowers physiological arousal and allows reframing to take hold.

When to Use It

When you're too activated to think clearly. Say: "I need 90 seconds," and walk away. Breathe. Come back calmer.

How it Integrates

The 90-second reset respects the body's design. God made emotions temporary if we don't rehearse them. Stepping away is trusting the body's natural regulation.

Tool 4: Confession Mirror

Isolation strengthens unhealthy emotional patterns. Bringing them into the light breaks their grip and invites correction.

What To Do

Once a week, meet with a trusted friend to confess one emotional misstep. Speak it plainly, receive correction, and rehearse a healthier response. This builds accountability and prevents hidden corrosion.

When To Use It

Weekly. Non-negotiable. This is the relational guardrail that keeps you honest.

How it Integrates

James 5:16 says the following:

"Confess your sins to one another and pray for one another, that you may be healed" (James 5:16).

Emotional dysregulation is sin when it damages relationships and dishonors God. Confession brings healing.

Tool 5: Prayer Integration

Emotional discipline is incomplete without surrender. Prayer brings your feelings under God's authority instead of your own.

What To Do

Name feelings honestly before God. State the reframe clearly, and ask for strength to live it out. This turns cognitive discipline into spiritual formation.

Here's an example: "God, I feel rejected. My friend didn't respond, and I'm telling myself I don't matter. But I know that's not true. My worth is rooted in you, not in response times. Help me believe that. Help me extend grace. Give me patience to wait without assuming the worst. Amen."

When To Use It

Daily. Especially in the morning and before bed. Bracket your day with honest prayer.

How it Integrates

Prayer is where emotional regulation becomes discipleship. You're not just managing feelings; you're aligning your heart with God's truth.

Tool 6: Scriptural Counterstatements

Lies often feel louder than truth. Scripture gives you language that counters deception and steadies your identity.

What To Do

Speak verses against embedded lies. Where the old story

says "I am worthless," Scripture declares "I am fearfully and wonderfully made" (Psalm 139:14). Where rejection says "I am alone," Scripture answers "I will never leave you nor forsake you" (Hebrews 13:5).

When To Use It

When lies feel louder than truth. Speak Scripture out loud. Let your ears hear it. Let your voice declare it.

How it Integrates

This is spiritual warfare. Lies are not just cognitive errors; they are spiritual attacks. Scripture is the sword (Ephesians 6:17). Use it.

Tool 7: Gratitude Practice

Attention shapes emotion. Deliberate gratitude retrains your focus and weakens envy, resentment, and anxiety.
Thanksgiving rewires attention away from scarcity.

What To Do

Name three specific gifts each day to shift your focus toward abundance and steadiness.

When To Use It

Daily. Morning or evening. Write them down. Be specific.
Example: Not "I'm thankful for my family" but "I'm thankful that my daughter laughed at dinner tonight."

How it Integrates

Gratitude is the antidote to envy and resentment. Philippians 4:6–7 connects thanksgiving to peace:

"Do not be anxious about anything, but in everything by prayer and supplication with thanksgiving let your requests be made known to God. And the peace of God . . . will guard your hearts" (Philippians 4:6–7).

THE PRINCIPLE

Small, repeatable moves compound into new defaults. When those moves are saturated with gospel truth, they reshape not only emotional response but spiritual posture.

These tools are not tricks. They are disciplines. They work because they align your interior life with the way God designed emotions to function: as signals to be stewarded, not tyrants to be obeyed or enemies to be suppressed.

PRACTICE PROMPT

❖ Every day for one week, pick one tool (micro-pause, one-sentence reframe, 90-second reset, or confession mirror). Use it once today in an ordinary moment.

❖ Then anchor it in prayer or Scripture: name the feeling before God, state the reframe, and thank Him for one gift connected to the moment.

❖ Write down how this integration changed your response.

Here's an example:

Today, I used the micro-pause when my coworker criticized my project. I named the feeling: hurt.

I asked, "What story am I telling?" The story was: "He thinks I'm incompetent."

I paused, breathed, and reframed: "He's giving feedback, not attacking me. I can receive it without defense."

Then I prayed: "God, I felt hurt. Thank you that my worth isn't tied to one person's opinion. Help me receive correction with humility."

I thanked God that I have work that matters. The hurt faded. I responded calmly.

Success Criteria

☐ You identified an EI gap (self-awareness, self-regulation, social awareness, or relationship management).

☐ You wrote one specific example of how that gap hurt you this week.

☐ You chose one practice to strengthen it, and implemented that practice for three out of seven days minimum.

Troubleshooting

If you couldn't identify a gap, you're overestimating your EI. Everyone has gaps. Ask someone close to you where they see your blind spots.

If you identified the gap but didn't practice, you're choosing comfort over growth.

If you practiced but saw no change, three days isn't enough. Keep going for thirty days before evaluating.

MARKERS OF PROGRESS

Training a sound heart is measurable. Progress is not abstract; it shows up in speech, relationships, and bodily steadiness. These markers help you discern whether the discipline is taking root.

Marker 1: Measured Speech

Responses slow down. You pause before speaking, allowing space for clarity instead of reaction.

Before, someone criticizes you. You snap back immediately.

After, someone criticizes you. You pause for five seconds. You name the feeling (hurt). You choose your words carefully: "I hear you. Let me think about that and respond tomorrow."

Expect this timeline: You might see this shift in two to three weeks of consistent practice.

Marker 2: Correction Received Without Defensiveness

Feedback no longer triggers immediate resistance. You can hear correction, weigh it, and adjust without corrosion.

Before, your spouse says, "You've been distant lately." You immediately defend: "I've been busy! What do you want from me?"

After, your spouse says, "You've been distant lately." You pause, name the feeling (shame), and respond: "You're right. I have been. I'm sorry. How can I do better?"

Expect this timeline: This often takes six to eight weeks to develop because defensiveness is deeply wired.

Marker 3: Celebration of Others Without Comparison

You rejoice in another's success without envy. The heart is steady enough to affirm others without self-diminishment.

Before, your friend gets promoted. You smile and congratulate them, but internally you're bitter. "Why not me?"

After, your friend gets promoted. You genuinely celebrate: "That's amazing! You earned this." And you mean it. The envy is gone.

Expect this timeline: This can take three to six months depending on how deeply comparison has been wired into your thinking.

Marker 4: Shortened Nighttime Loops

Rumination at night decreases. Sleep improves as emotional charge is reduced and reframes take hold.

Before, you lie awake replaying a conversation for two hours. "I should have said this. Why did I say that?"

After, you replay the conversation once, reframe it ("I did my best. I can address it tomorrow if needed"), and fall asleep within twenty minutes.

Expect this timeline: Often four to six weeks brings change. Better sleep is one of the first physical signs that emotional regulation is working.

Marker 5: Faster Repair in Relationships

Conflict still happens, but repair comes more quickly. Apologies are offered sooner, reconciliation is pursued more directly.

Before, you have a fight with your spouse. You stew for three days. Eventually, you apologize, but the damage lingers.

After, you have a fight with your spouse. Within two hours, you come back: "I was harsh. I'm sorry. Can we talk?" Repair happens before bitterness sets in.

Expect this timeline: It's often two to four months. This requires both emotional regulation and relational skill.

Marker 6: Tracking High-Stress Episodes

One practical measure: note one high-stress episode each week. Record your response. Over time, the notes reveal shorter recovery windows, steadier speech, and healthier reframes.

PRACTICE PROMPT

- ❖ Keep a simple log:
    - Date
    - Trigger
    - Initial emotion
    - Response (what I said/did)
    - Reframe (if applicable)

- ❖ After four weeks, review. You'll see progress even when it doesn't feel like progress in the moment.

Realistic Timelines

Don't expect immediate mastery. Progress can be measured like this:

- **Weeks one through three:** Increased awareness. You're catching emotions earlier.
- **Weeks four through eight:** Slower reactions. You're pausing more consistently.
- **Months three through six:** Visible change. Others notice you're calmer, less reactive.
- **Months six through twelve:** New defaults. The practices become automatic.

This is a marathon, not a sprint. Celebrate small wins.

PRACTICE PROMPT

- ❖ For the next month, keep a simple progress journal. Each week, record one high-stress episode and how you responded.

- ❖ At the end of the month, review the entries and identify which markers of progress are most evident.

Week one:

- Episode: Coworker criticized my work in front of team.
- Emotion: Embarrassment, angerResponse: I snapped back defensively.
- Reframe: I later reframed it ("He's stressed about the deadline, not attacking me."), but damage was done.
- Marker: I'm not yet seeing measured speech.

Week four:

- Episode: A coworker criticized my work in front of team.
- Emotion: Embarrassment (I caught it early.)
- Response: I paused, named it, and said, "Thanks for the feedback. Let's discuss details after the meeting."
- Reframe: "His feedback is data. I can use it to improve."
- Marker: Measured speech is showing up!

Success Criteria

□ You chose two tools from the section (breath work, body scan, name-and-claim, journaling, or prayer).
□ You used both tools daily for seven consecutive days.
□ You journaled after each use, noting what you observed about your emotional state.

Troubleshooting

If you used them a few times then quit, you're treating tools like inspiration instead of discipline. Tools work through repetition, not novelty.

If one tool isn't working, don't abandon it after two uses. Give it a full week before deciding.

If both tools feel useless, you're not engaging honestly with your emotions during the practice. Slow down, and actually feel what's there.

FINAL NOTES AND WARNINGS

Emotional training is lifelong work. A sound heart is not achieved by one breakthrough but by steady rehearsal. These final notes guard against common missteps and set expectations for the journey.

Warning 1: Don't stop at naming.

Labeling emotions is only the first step. Without movement through the full sequence (Name → Accept → Analyze → Express → Reframe), naming alone becomes stagnation.

You can name anger all day long. If you never express it in a healthy way or reframe it toward truth, you're just rehearsing the feeling without moving it.

The fix: Commit to the full sequence. Name is the entry point, not the destination.

Warning 2: Don't spiritualize avoidance.

Quoting Scripture or praying without facing the emotion honestly is evasion, not integration. Spiritual practices must be paired with truthful engagement, not used as a shield against discomfort.

Example: You're angry at your spouse. Instead of addressing it, you pray, "God, help me be more patient." You never tell your spouse what hurt you. The anger festers. That's not spiritual maturity; it's avoidance disguised as piety.

The fix is to pray honestly ("God, I'm angry at my spouse for [specific thing]"), then address it directly with the person.

Warning 3: Don't weaponize labels.

Emotional vocabulary is meant for stewardship, not attack. Using labels to shame or control others corrodes relationships and undermines the discipline.

Example: "You're being envious." "You're just insecure." "That's your anxiety talking."

When you use EI to diagnose and dismiss others, you've turned a tool into a weapon.

The fix is to use labels on yourself. Let others name their own emotions. Offer observation, not diagnosis: "I noticed you seemed tense. Are you okay?"

Warning 4: Don't expect immediate mastery.

This is lifelong rehearsal. Progress is measured in shortened loops, steadier speech, and quicker repair, not perfection. Expect setbacks, but treat them as training opportunities.

Here's a reality check: You'll still snap sometimes. You'll still ruminate. You'll still defend. That's normal. The question is: how quickly do you recover? Are the episodes getting less frequent? Less intense? Shorter?

The fix is to track progress over months, not days. Compare yourself to yourself six months ago, not to some ideal version you imagine.

Warning 5: Having a weekly review plus an accountability partner is essential.

Without review and community, the practice drifts. A weekly check-in with a trusted partner keeps the discipline sharp and prevents hidden corrosion.

It matters because you lie to yourself. You always have. You always will. An external voice catches what you miss.

The fix is to schedule a weekly 15-minute call or coffee with your accountability partner. Share one emotional misstep. Rehearse a healthier response. Ask for feedback.

PRACTICE PROMPT

❖ Identify one person you trust to walk with you in this disciplineShare one emotional misstep from the past week and rehearse a healthier response together.

❖ Record the conversation in your journal as part of your weekly review.

Example:

This week, I snapped at my kid when they interrupted me during work. I felt disrespected, but I didn't pause. I just reacted.

With my accountability partner, I rehearsed: Next time, I'll name the feeling (disrespected), take a breath, and say calmly, "I need you to wait until I'm done with this call, please." Then I'll follow up after the call to reconnect.

My partner asked, "Are you willing to apologize to your kid for snapping?" I said yes. I did it that night. It felt hard, but it was right.

Success Criteria

☐ You rated yourself on all six markers (fewer reactive moments, better sleep, clearer thinking, stronger relationships, increased patience, and a more peaceful presence).
☐ You identified your weakest marker.
☐ You wrote one specific action to improve it.
☐ You implemented that action for the week.
☐ You rated yourself again seven days later to measure change.

Troubleshooting

If all your ratings are high but people around you would disagree, you're grading yourself on intention, not impact. Ask someone close to you to rate you instead.

If your weakest marker didn't improve after a week, either your action was too vague or you didn't actually do it consistently. Be honest about which one.

CONCLUSION

A sound heart is both trainable and necessary. It is not a gift reserved for the few but a discipline available to all who commit to the sequence.

Sequence Recap

The path is clear:

Name → Accept → Analyze → Express → Reframe.

Each step builds on the other, forming a complete system for emotional regulation. This is not theory. This is the practical, repeatable method for training emotions so they serve you instead of ruling you.

Memorize the sequence. Write it down. Post it where you'll see it daily. Let it become second nature.

Emotional Intelligence as the Engine

Emotional intelligence provides the deeper skills that make the sequence effective—perceiving, understanding, and managing emotions with precision. It is the engine that drives the practice forward.

Without EI, the sequence stalls. With EI, it becomes reflexive.

Spiritual Anchors

Prayer, Scripture, and community saturate the process with gospel truth. Without these anchors, reframing risks becoming self-management. With them, it becomes spiritual growth, guarding the heart and renewing the mind.

We are not talking about secular psychology with a Bible verse slapped on. This is discipleship—the daily work of conforming your inner life to the character of Christ.

Fruit of the Discipline

The outcomes are tangible:

- **Life to the body.** Lower cortisol. Better sleep. Stronger immunity. Longer lifespan.
- **Clarity to the mind.** Sharper thinking. Better decisions. Resistance to manipulation.
- **Steadiness in relationships.** Faster repair. Less defensiveness. More patience.
- **Resilience in witness and work.** You can serve longer, lead better, and love more consistently.

A sound heart produces a life that lasts.

PRACTICE PROMPT

❖ Begin today with one micro move—a pause, a reframe, or a prayer. Pair it with one accountability conversation this week.

Progress is not measured in perfection but in steady rehearsal. Show up. Do the work. Notice the change.

The Stakes

This is not optional. Your heart shapes everything downstream. That's is why it is first stop in The SCAL Method.

Your speech. Your decisions. Your relationships. Your witness.

Your health. Your longevity. Your capacity to serve. An unsound heart corrodes all of it. A sound heart sustains all of it.

So guard your heart. Train it. Steward it daily. The fruit will be life—for you, for your relationships, for your witness, and for the generations that come after you.

CHAPTER TWO
A SOUND MIND

"For God hath not given us the spirit of fear; but of power, and of love, and of a sound mind" (2 Timothy 1:7).

UNDERSTANDING A SOUND MIND

Years ago, I worked at UPS as a package sorter. It was honest work, grabbing packages and routing them down conveyor belts, shift after shift. I was young, clean-shaven, and most days, I looked more exhausted than the older workers around me. One man in particular stood out. He was in his early fifties, methodical, never rushed, and always seemed to have energy left when everyone else was running on fumes.

We'd talk during breaks, and our conversations always drifted toward philosophy, who we wanted to become, what we were working toward, the kind of men we hoped to be.

On one of my last shifts before moving on, he said something that didn't register at the time. He called me "a sound thinker." It wasn't something he said as a throwaway statement. He meant it. At least, that's how I interpreted his insistence that I listen to him when he said it.

I thanked him politely and kept moving, but the weight of that compliment didn't hit me until years later.

"Sound" doesn't sound like much. It's not flashy. It doesn't draw attention. But when you understand what it means, steady, reliable, free from damage, not easily shaken, you realize it's one of the highest compliments you can give or receive. A sound individual is someone whose mind holds under pressure, whose judgment doesn't waver with mood, whose decisions can be trusted. That man saw something in me I was still building. His words stuck because they named a target worth aiming for.

Part two of the SCAL Method

The second part of the SCAL method is having a sound mind. We're going to run three basic questions and then get down to the work: What is a sound mind? Why do you want one? How do you train to get one? I must forewarn you that this process isn't particularly a fun one; this is quiet work, the kind people avoid because it's slower and harder than chasing feelings and instant validation, but it's the work that wins.

Paul's line to Timothy is a job order. Timothy was shy, unsure, and now charged with carrying the work forward. Paul's point is simple and to the point: don't be scared. The Spirit gives you power, love, and mental sobriety. Stand on business because the Spirit is in you.

Translation

The Greek behind "sound mind" is *sōphronismos,* a word that lands closer to meaning disciplined, self-controlled, and levelheaded than to cleverness or IQ. Lexical sources show it's used exactly once in the New Testament, in this verse, carrying that sense of moderation, self-control, and practical sobriety. Lexicons parse it as "self-control" and "moderation," and they tie it to words meaning to be safe-minded or apt to act sensibly in a situation. It's not academic vocabulary reserved for the lecture hall but a working term for a person who keeps their head in heat and decisions in line.

That's the setup. That's the standard. A sound mind is not saying you should be devoid of emotion. Rather, it's the personal trainer for your heart. It notices the pull of a feeling, names it, and then either lets it drive action or puts it on the bench depending on what the situation needs.

When you build this capacity, you stop suffering the cheap, predictable wreckage of reaction. You make better decisions, resist manipulation., and compound good outcomes across generations.

This chapter gives you the framework, the practices, and the rationale. The verse is your commission. The work is yours to do.

HOW THIS CONNECTS

A sound mind doesn't work in isolation. It's the training ground for discernment that strengthens every other arena:

- **Sound Heart:** The mind reframes destructive thoughts and challenges emotional distortions. Train the mind, and the heart steadies. Mental clarity interrupts anxiety spirals and keeps feelings from hijacking judgment.

- **Strong Body:** Physical discipline requires planning, strategy, and delayed gratification. A trained mind makes better decisions about rest, nutrition, and training intensity. Mental laziness leads to inconsistent effort and wasted potential.

- **Strong Soul:** Mental clarity creates space for prayer, contemplation, and discernment. You can't seek God's wisdom if your mind is cluttered with noise. A sound mind distinguishes truth from deception and anchors spiritual practices in reality.

A sound mind produces discernment. An unsound mind breeds confusion. What governs the mind ripples outward into relationships, decisions, and legacy.

VERSE, CONTEXT, AND WORD

Paul wrote this near the end of his life, passing the baton to a younger man. Timothy was shy, prone to shrinking, and now charged with carrying the work forward without Paul standing beside him. The instruction is direct: the Spirit living in you is not a spirit of fear. He gives power, love, and mental sobriety.

Walk like it.

The Greek word behind "sound mind" is sōphronismos, appearing exactly once in the New Testament, right here in this verse. Lexical sources render it as self-control, moderation, and safe-mindedness —the quality of a person who stays steady under pressure and acts sensibly when others lose their footing. This is not a word for academic brilliance or raw intelligence. It describes someone who keeps their head when the heat is on and keeps their decisions in line when emotion is pulling hard. Understanding what "sound mind" means in Greek is one thing. Seeing what it looks like when lived is another.

A sound mind is not just an abstract quality or spiritual ideal; it's a functional capacity that shapes every decision, conversation, and response. Let's break down how it actually operates in daily life.

A SOUND MIND SOUNDS LIKE

A sound mind is not emotionless. It's not a cold, dead thing. It's the personal trainer for your heart. A sound mind notices the pull of a feeling, names it, and then either lets it drive action or puts it on the bench depending on what the situation needs.

Think of the decision flow like this: perceive the data, comprehend what that likely means, evaluate with judgment, then decide and act. When each of those steps is sharp, outcomes are useful and stable; when any one is sloppy, you wreck your own life and the lives of the people who depend on you.

A sound mind sharpens perception, tightens evaluation, and disciplines action so you don't suffer the cheap, predictable wreckage of reaction.

Nobody is born with a sound mind fully formed. It's muscle and skill. It's trained by sitting still, testing your thinking, and getting merciless about the things that keep you small.

Real-World Example: Jade Receives a Critical Email

Jade receives an email from her boss criticizing a project she worked hard on. The words feel harsh. Her heart rate spikes. Here's how two different versions of Jade handle the exact same situation.

Unsound Mind Jade perceives the situation as "He attacked me." She interprets critique as personal assault. She comprehends the email to mean "He doesn't value my work. He thinks I'm incompetent," jumping immediately to worst-case meaning. Her evaluation is driven entirely by emotion: "This is unfair. I need to defend myself." Within minutes, she fires off a defensive reply, escalating the conflict.

Sound Mind Jade perceives the same email differently: "He sent critical feedback about the project." Accurate, emotion-neutral observation. She comprehends it as "He's identifying specific areas that didn't meet expectations," sticking to the data.

Her evaluation is rational: "Some points are valid. Some may be misunderstandings. I should clarify before responding."

She waits an hour, rereads the email, asks clarifying questions, then responds professionally with a plan to address legitimate concerns.

Same situation. Different outcomes.

Unsound Mind Jade created conflict, damaged the relationship, and learned nothing.

Sound Mind Jade preserved the relationship, identified real problems, and grew.

That pause between stimulus and response is where a sound mind operates.

Seeing how a sound mind operates in real time clarifies what's at stake. But understanding the mechanics isn't enough.

You need to know why cultivating this capacity matters, not just for your own well-being, but for everyone whose life intersects with yours.

A sound mind is not a personal luxury; it's a generational responsibility.

PRACTICE PROMPT

- ❖ Pick one situation from the last 24 hours where you felt an emotional spike: frustration, anger, anxiety, excitement.

- ❖ Write out what you actually perceived versus what you told yourself it meant.

❖ Answer these questions: Where did emotion hijack the flow? What would the sound mind version do differently?

Success Criteria

☐ You identified one specific emotional spike from the last twenty-four hours.
☐ You separated facts from interpretation.
☐ You spotted where emotion hijacked your response.
☐ You described what a sound mind would have done.
☐ You practiced the thirty-second pause for three consecutive days.

Troubleshooting

If you can't remember an emotional spike, you're not paying attention. Notice physical cues: tight chest, clenched jaw, racing heart.

If you can't separate perception from interpretation, slow down.

Facts: "He sent critical feedback."

Interpretation: "He thinks I'm incompetent."

If your response already looks sound, consider whether you're lying to yourself.

WHY YOU WANT A SOUND MIND

You want a sound mind because it does three things no one and nothing else will do for you consistently: it keeps your emotions in check, it immunizes you against manipulation, and it compounds better choices into a legacy for the people who come after you. Emotions are informative but undisciplined; a trained mind turns them into reliable data instead of a tyrant. A sound mind asks, "Who benefits?" and "What evidence?" before swallowing a headline or someone else's noise driven reaction. That resistance to manipulation is not cynicism; it's survival. When decisions are made with clear perception, careful evaluation, and moral purpose, good outcomes compound across households and communities; the micro-decisions of daily life scale into macro results that affect generations.

And because we have this set up in this way where you perceive, comprehend, you make a judgment, *then* you make a decision, a sound mind cannot be manipulated. I repeat, a sound mind cannot be manipulated.

Real-World Example: Jade and the Viral Post

Jade scrolls past a shocking headline: "BREAKING: New Study Proves [Thing She Dislikes] Is Dangerous!"

The post has 50,000 shares, hundreds of angry comments, and urgent language designed to provoke immediate sharing.

Here's how the two versions of Jade respond.

Unsound Mind Jade

Unsound Mind Jade feels an instant emotional spike: fear, anger, validation. She shares immediately without reading past the headline. She doesn't ask who wrote this, what their motive might be, or what the actual study says. She becomes an amplifier for potentially false or misleading information.

The neurotransmitter hit of righteous outrage feels like truth, but it's just reaction.

Sound Mind Jade

Sound Mind Jade notices the same emotional spike and names it: "I'm feeling activated." She pauses.

Then she asks, "What's the source? Who funded the study? Is this peer-reviewed?" She looks for two independent confirmations from credible sources. She asks, "Who benefits if I believe this? What would change my mind?"

After checking, she either confirms and shares with context, or she ignores it as unverified.

This isn't paranoia or obstinacy. It's discernment.

Unsound Mind Jade is an easy target for manipulation because she reacts instead of responds.

Sound Mind Jade resists manipulation because she inserts friction, pause, questions, verification, before belief or action. In an age of information warfare, this isn't optional. It's survival.

A sound mind gives you capacity, the ability to perceive,

evaluate, and decide well. But capacity alone isn't enough.

You also need direction. You need to know what's worth pursuing and what's worth avoiding. That's where wisdom enters.

Wisdom is the moral and spiritual intelligence that guides a sound mind toward truth and away from clever destruction. Without wisdom, a sharp mind can be weaponized. With wisdom, a sharp mind becomes a tool for flourishing.

PRACTICE PROMPT

❖ Think of something you recently believed, shared, or acted on quickly: a social media post, a news story, or a conversation that made you angry or afraid. Then run it through these questions:
- Did it create urgency? ("Share this now!")
- Did it trigger strong emotion immediately? (outrage, fear, validation)
- Did it oversimplify a complex issue into good vs. evil?
- Did you verify it with two independent sources before believing/sharing?
- Did it confirm what you already wanted to believe?

If you answered yes to three or more, you were likely manipulated.

❖ Write which step in the decision flow got hijacked. Did you skip perception (didn't check facts)? Comprehension (accepted the first meaning)? Evaluation (let emotion decide)?

Success Criteria

☐ You identified one recent belief/action and ran it through the five manipulation questions.

☐ You determined whether you were manipulated (3+ yes answers).

☐ You traced which decision step was hijacked.

☐ For one week, you asked, "Who benefits?" and "What would change my mind?" before acting on emotionally charged information.

Troubleshooting

If you answered no to all five questions, you're either unusually discerning or lying to yourself. Most people get manipulated on a regular basis.

If you can't identify any recent beliefs that triggered emotion, check your social media. It's designed to trigger you.

If asking "Who benefits?" feels paranoid, that discomfort is the sound mind waking up. Stay with it.

TO FEAR NOT

Fear gets a bad rap in Christian circles. We hear "fear not" somewhere around 365 times in Scripture, depending on the translation. That's one for every day of the year, and we conclude that fear itself is the enemy. That's sloppy thinking.

Fear is an emotion. Like anger, grief, and joy, fear is part of the human design. The problem isn't fear. The problem is what you do with it.

Healthy fear is protective. Fear of a cliff edge keeps you from walking off. Fear of fire keeps your hand out of the flame. Fear of consequences can prevent foolish decisions. That's fear doing what it was designed to do: signal danger, preserve life, create caution where caution is warranted.

The issue is when fear becomes your operating system, when it stops being a signal and starts being your master. When it distorts your perception, hijacks your judgment, and drives your decisions, that's when fear becomes destructive. And that's what Paul is addressing when he tells Timothy, "God hath not given us the spirit of fear."

Courage Requiring Fear

Here's something most people miss: you cannot have courage without fear. Courage is not the absence of fear. It's the decision to act rightly in spite of fear. You can't be brave about something that doesn't scare you. That's just called doing a normal thing.

Joshua wasn't told, "Don't be afraid" because he wasn't afraid. He was told, "Be strong and of a good courage; be not afraid, neither be thou dismayed: for the Lord thy God is with thee whithersoever thou goest" (Joshua 1:9) precisely because he had every reason to be afraid. He was leading an entire nation into enemy territory. The fear was real. The courage was the choice to obey anyway.

Jesus didn't tell his disciples, "Be of good cheer" (Matthew 9:2, John 16:33) because they were naturally gloomy. He said it because they were terrified. The storms were real. The persecution was coming. The fear made sense. But Jesus gave them something stronger than the fear: himself. "Be of good cheer; I have overcome the world" (John 16:33). The cheer wasn't denial. It was defiance grounded in truth.

Courage is trained emotional regulation applied to fear. It's the ability to feel the fear, name it, analyze it, and then choose the right action anyway. That's a sound mind in operation.

The Spirit of Fear

Let's go back to the anchor verse. It says, "For God hath not given us the spirit of fear; but of power, and of love, and of a sound mind" (2 Timothy 1:7).

Paul isn't saying God didn't create the emotion of fear. He's saying God didn't give you a spirit of fear. What's the difference?

"Spirit of" in Scripture refers to a ruling disposition, a habitual pattern, the thing you consistently do. It's not a one-time occurrence. It's a way of being. Look at how Scripture uses this phrase elsewhere:

- **Romans 8:15** says, "For ye have not received the spirit of bondage again to fear; but ye have received the spirit of adoption, whereby we cry, Abba, Father." Consider the spirit of bondage versus spirit of adoption. One is a pattern of slavery. The other is a pattern of belonging.

- **1 Corinthians 2:12** says, "Now we have received not the spirit of the world but the Spirit which is of God." Contrast the spirit of the world versus the Spirit of God. They are two different operating systems, two different patterns of thinking and living.

- **Isaiah 61:3** says that God gives "the garment of praise for the spirit of heaviness." Spirit of heaviness isn't occasional sadness. It's a crushing, chronic weight. The garment of praise is the antidote.

- **Galatians 6:1** says, "Restore such an one in the spirit of meekness." Spirit of meekness is how you habitually approach correction: gently, humbly, with care.

See the pattern? "Spirit of" describes your default mode, your habitual response, the thing you consistently return to.

So when Paul says God hasn't given you the spirit of fear, he's not saying you'll never feel afraid. He's saying fear doesn't have to be your default setting. Fear doesn't get to be the thing that rules your perception, your decisions, your life.

Instead, God gave you the spirit of power, love, and a sound mind. Power to act. Love to guide action. A sound mind to discern when and how.

How Fear Distorts the Decision Flow

Here's where it gets practical. Remember the decision sequence:

$$\text{Perceive} \rightarrow \text{Comprehend} \rightarrow \text{Evaluate} \rightarrow \text{Decide} \rightarrow \text{Act}$$

A sound mind moves through these steps with clarity and precision. Fear scrambles every single one.

Fear distorts perception. You see threats that aren't there. You magnify danger and minimize resources. A critical email becomes a personal attack. A financial setback becomes total ruin. Fear narrows your vision and amplifies the negative.

Fear warps comprehension. Even if you perceive correctly, fear twists the meaning. "He gave me feedback" becomes "He thinks I'm incompetent and wants me gone." Fear fills gaps with worst-case interpretations.

Fear corrupts evaluation. Under fear, judgment collapses. You can't weigh evidence objectively. You can't ask, "What's actually true here?" because fear has already decided the answer. Everything confirms the threat.

Fear paralyzes decision. Even when you know what's right, fear freezes you. You hesitate. You procrastinate. You convince yourself you need more information. You never have enough courage to act because fear keeps moving the threshold.

Fear sabotages action. If you do act, fear makes it reactive and sloppy. You lash out. You run. You defend when you should listen. You escalate when you should pause.

The spirit of fear is a wrecking ball for sound thinking. It corrodes discernment, breeds anxiety, and produces outcomes you'll regret. That's why training your mind is not optional. You're in a fight, and fear is the weapon your enemy uses to keep you small, reactive, and ineffective.

The training that follows isn't theoretical. Well, a lot of theory did go into this, but it's even more a practical method for breaking fear's grip on your decision-making and building the mental discipline that turns fear from a master into a signal you can evaluate and act on with wisdom.

GROUNDWORK AND SEQUENCE

A sound mind is not an accident. It's built through deliberate practice. Training your mind requires systematic work across four areas, each one corresponding to a step in the decision flow you learned earlier. This training sharpens your mind the way a whetstone sharpens a blade.

How a Sound Mind Processes Decisions

Every decision you make follows a sequence:

$$\text{Perceive} \to \text{Comprehend} \to \text{Evaluate} \to \text{Decide} \to \text{Act}$$

Training a sound mind means strengthening each step in this chain:

Perceive: Observe the data accurately without distortion.

Comprehend: Understand what the data means.

Evaluate: Judge whether conclusions are supported by evidence.

Decide: Choose a course of action.

Act: Execute the decision.

When each step is sharp, outcomes are useful and stable. When any one is sloppy, you wreck your own life and the lives of people who depend on you. The four training areas below target each part of this sequence.

1. Perception Training

Perception is the foundation. If you perceive incorrectly, then everything downstream fails. Most people don't observe — they project. They see what they want to see, what they expect to see, or what they fear. Perception training means observing the data as it actually is, not as you wish it to be.

The goal is accurate observation without immediate interpretation.

The result is that you stop reacting to interpretations and start responding to reality.

2. Comprehension Training

Comprehension is where you move from raw observation to meaning-making. This step asks, "What does this information tell me? What patterns exist? What's the context?"

Without strong comprehension, you'll either miss what matters or jump to conclusions that aren't supported.

The goal is understanding what the data actually means.

The result is that you understand what's actually happening instead of what you think is happening. You catch nuance, context, and meaning that others miss.

3. Evaluation Training

Evaluation is where you assess the quality of your comprehension and decide if it's trustworthy. This step asks: "Is this true? What's the evidence? What would change my mind?"

Strong evaluation separates reliable conclusions from wishful thinking.

The goal is having sound judgment about whether conclusions are supported.

The result is that your judgments become reliable. You can separate truth from manipulation, signal from noise, and solid conclusions from emotional reactions.

4. Decision Training

A sound mind that never acts is useless. Decision training is where perception, comprehension, and evaluation converge into movement. This step trains you to decide without paralysis and act without recklessness.

The goal is taking decisive action based on sound evaluation.

The result is that you become a person of action. Your decisions are grounded, your execution is confident, and you don't second-guess yourself into paralysis.

HOW AREAS WORK TOGETHER

These four training areas aren't separate practices. They form a cycle. Each step strengthens the others:

Perception training gives you clean data → Comprehension training helps you understand what it means → Evaluation training tests whether your understanding is sound → Decision training turns evaluation into movement.

Then the cycle repeats. Each decision teaches you to perceive more accurately next time.

Example: The Training Cycle in Action

Scenario: You're offered a new job.

- **Perception:** Write down the facts. They might include things liks salary, responsibilities, location, team size. No interpretation happens yet.

- **Comprehension:** What does this opportunity mean? How does it align with your long-term goals? What's the context of this offer within the company and industry?

- **Evaluation:** Research the company. Talk to current employees. Ask, "What's the evidence this is a good fit? What's the evidence it's not?" Pray for wisdom. Read Proverbs 16:3, which says, "Commit thy works unto the Lord, and thy thoughts shall be established."

- **Decision:** Make the call. Accept or decline. Don't waffle. Don't second-guess. Trust the process.

The training gives you confidence because you've practiced each step. The decision might still be hard, but it won't be reckless or paralyzed.

HOW ONE STRENGTHENS ALL

Sound Heart

A trained mind regulates emotions. Perception and comprehension give your heart the data it needs to respond appropriately instead of reactively.

Strong Body

Decision training builds decisiveness, which carries into physical discipline. A mind that executes decisions doesn't procrastinate workouts.

Strong Soul

Evaluation training deepens your spiritual life. Integrating wisdom into evaluation trains you to hear God's voice, which strengthens prayer, Scripture reading, and spiritual discernment.

A sound mind is the personal trainer for your heart, the strategist for your body, and the steward of your soul.

WHAT CRITICAL THINKING IS

First off, let's lock down a working definition you can carry into every conversation and decision: critical thinking is the disciplined work of collecting reliable information and then doing the hard, sometimes boring analytic labor to turn that information into a trustworthy decision.

If you want the longer academic formulation so you know you're arguing from somewhere recognized, see Michael Scriven and Richard Paul's definition. It captures the structure, an intellectually disciplined process of actively and skillfully conceptualizing, applying, analyzing, synthesizing, and evaluating information gathered from observation, experience, reflection, reasoning, or communication.

Now, say that five times fast. That's a lot. It also sounds like a lot of work, and it is. It's intellectual work. To beef up your critical thinking skills, you have to work.

The basis of critical thinking is collecting then analyzing. And a number of different things branch out from under those two subsets of critical thinking. But the idea is to accrue skills that make you better at those two practices.

Critical thinking trains the first two steps of the framework: **perception and comprehension.** Collection sharpens your ability to perceive accurately—gathering clean data without distortion. Analysis strengthens comprehension—understanding what that data actually means and whether it's reliable.

Without these foundational skills, every subsequent step fails. You can't evaluate what you don't understand, and you can't understand what you haven't accurately observed.

These sections give you the tools to build a reliable foundation for every decision you make.

PRACTICE PROMPT

- ❖ Pick one thing you believe strongly—about politics, health, relationships, money, anything. Write it down.

- ❖ Now, write where this belief came from. (Was it a person? An article? One experience? Something you grew up hearing?)

- ❖ Then ask yourself, "Did I ever test this belief, or did I just accept it?"

- ❖ Find one source that disagrees with your belief. Read it. Write one sentence: "They argue that [X]."

Success Criteria

☐ You identified one specific belief and traced where it came from.

☐ You assessed whether you tested it or just accepted it.

☐ You found a source that disagrees.

☐ You wrote their main argument in one sentence.

Troubleshooting

If you can't think of a belief, pick something you'd defend in an argument or something you'd feel uncomfortable questioning. If everything you believe came from careful testing, pick your most recent strong opinion and trace it anyway.

If you can't find a disagreeing source, you're filtering your search. Try: "Why [your belief] is wrong."

If reading the disagreement made you angry, notice that reaction. It reveals how much your identity is tied to the belief.

CRITICAL THINKING: COLLECTING

Start with collection, because without decent raw material, your analysis is garbage. Collection is not passive scrolling or grabbing the easiest headline that confirms your mood; collection is active listening, disciplined research, and high-quality observation done deliberately so you have the right inputs to test.

Active listening looks like shutting up long enough to map what the other person is actually saying and then summarizing it back before you respond so you know you heard them instead of your echo chamber. In practice, this means holding genuine curiosity about why someone arrived at their position rather than mentally rehearsing your rebuttal while they speak.

Research means deliberately hunting for the strongest arguments against your position as well as the strongest evidence for it. Track origins, prioritize sources that show methods and data, and mark secondary summaries as what they are. Know when to stop collecting. Once you've found both strong support and credible objections and you understand the methodological quality of each source, adding more sources becomes procrastination.

Observation is the slow work of noticing micro-data: cadence shifts, recurring language, body language that contradicts words, patterns in behavior that outlast a single heat-of-the-moment claim. This skill develops through repetition: start by watching one conversation per week without participating, noting three specific behavioral patterns you wouldn't have caught if you were talking. Over time, you'll begin noticing these patterns in real time, which lets you separate performance from genuine belief.

These three skills work together: listening captures what people actually say, research validates claims with evidence, and observation reveals patterns that words alone might hide.

Turn collection into habit with cheap rituals: ten minutes of focused reading from a robust long-form piece, then ten minutes listing the three best counter-arguments; do that three times a week and you'll shift from noisy accumulation to selective, testable intake.

Example of Poor vs. Strong Collection
Topic: Should I change my diet?
Poor Collection

- Scrolls Instagram, sees fitness influencer promoting a carnivore diet.
- Watches one YouTube video titled "Carnivore Cured My Problems!"
- Asks one friend who also just started carnivore.
- Decides based on three sources that all confirm the same thing.

Strong Collection

- Reads peer-reviewed studies on carnivore diets (not just abstracts, actual methodology).
- Actively seeks critiques: "What are the downsides of carnivore?" "Who shouldn't do carnivore?"
- Talks to a registered dietitian (expert, not influencer).
- Observes own body's signals: energy levels, sleep quality, workout performance.
- Tracks origins: Who funded the studies promoting carnivore? What's the influencer selling?

The difference is intentionality. Poor collection accepts whatever confirms the impulse. Strong collection hunts for disconfirming evidence and prioritizes credible sources over convenient ones.

PRACTICE PROMPT

- ❖ Pick one collecting skill to practice this week:
  - Active Listening—In one conversation, just listen. Don't plan your response. Map what they're actually saying. After, write down what you heard.
  - Research—Pick one topic you disagree with. Find the strongest arguments for it. Write down the best one.
  - Observation—Watch someone for five minutes without speaking. Write what you noticed about their body language, tone, patterns.

- ❖ Do this three times this week with the same skill.

Success Criteria

☐ You chose one collecting skill.
☐ You practiced it three times this week.
☐ You wrote down what you noticed each time.

Troubleshooting

If you chose active listening but kept planning your response, your mind is too loud. Try again, and focus only on their words.

If you researched but couldn't find strong arguments for the opposing view, you're searching with bias. Add "best case for" to your search.

If you observed but saw nothing worth noting, you're not slowing down enough. Watch for micro-expressions, hand movements, voice changes.

If you only did it once instead of three times, pick a smaller time commitment. Try two minutes instead of five.

Critical Thinking: Analyzing

Collection alone won't save you. Analysis is the heavy lifting and where most people fall apart. Analysis rests on three habits you must actually practice: ruthless self-awareness, relentless curiosity, and steady judgment.

Self-awareness is the brutal but clarifying work of naming your priors before you ever evaluate evidence: write down what you already believe and why, then list the emotional or social levers that make those beliefs comfortable. Without this step, you'll mistake confirmation bias for careful thinking, cherry-picking evidence that supports conclusions you've already emotionally committed to.

Curiosity means disciplined interrogation. Ask, "What evidence would change my mind?" and "What would the best objection say?" The goal is to stress-test your position by actively seeking the single strongest counter-argument that could actually threaten your conclusion.

Judgment is procedural closure: a calibrated decision about whether available data supports a tentative conclusion and how uncertain you remain. Strong judgment means knowing when you have enough information to act, assigning realistic confidence levels to your conclusions, and staying honest about what you don't know rather than inflating certainty to feel secure.

Analysis only works when all three habits operate together: self-awareness catches your biases, curiosity tests your reasoning, and judgment decides when thinking becomes doing.

Train these by keeping a short nightly log: what belief did I test today, what did I find, and why might someone reasonable disagree with my read? After a month, you'll have a mirror for blind spots and a record you can query later.

Don't treat these three habits like slogans. Make them operational. For self-awareness, build a checklist that names incentives and identity stakes: whose money, reputation, or belonging benefits if I keep this belief? For curiosity, develop a set of disconfirming prompts, such as "What would have to be false for this claim to collapse," and practice them out loud until they feel normal. For judgment, create a one-paragraph template you use on any significant claim. State the claim, list supporting evidence, list the strongest countering evidence, give a confidence tag (low/medium/high), and identify one experiment or check that could move your confidence.

Example of an Analysis Template in Action

Claim: "Intermittent fasting (IF) is the best way to lose weight."

Self-Awareness Check:
What do I already believe? I want a simple solution. I'm tired of counting calories.
Who benefits if I believe this? The influencer selling a fasting course. My ego (I can feel smart for finding the "secret").

Curiosity Questions
What evidence would change my mind? Studies showing fasting has no metabolic advantage over calorie matching.
What would the best objection say? "Fasting works for some but isn't universal. Adherence matters more than method."

Supporting Evidence Review: Some studies show weight loss with IF. Anecdotal success stories.

Countering Evidence Review: Meta-analyses show IF and continuous calorie restriction produce similar results when calories are matched. Adherence varies by individual.

Judgment: The original claim is too absolute. Intermittent fasting is a viable weight-loss method for many people, but the evidence doesn't crown it the best — it crowns consistency.

Confidence: Medium. Intermittent fasting is one effective method for weight loss, but not universally "the best." Success depends on adherence.

Experiment: Try it for 30 days while tracking calories, energy, and adherence. Compare to a non-IF approach for 30 days. Measure results.

This template forces honesty. It prevents jumping from "I want this to be true" to "This is definitely true."

Understanding how to collect and analyze data is one thing. Building the habit of doing it consistently is another. Knowledge without repetition stays theoretical. You need to turn these skills into reflexes, patterns that activate automatically when you encounter information, decisions, or arguments. That's where the habit-building work begins.

PRACTICE PROMPT

❖ Choose one piece of information you accepted recently — a news headline, advice from a friend, something you saw online, something you heard in church.

❖ Run it through this analysis grid, writing your answers to all four:
  • What are my biases around this? (What do I want to be true?)
  • What questions should I ask? (Who benefits? What's missing?)
  • Is the source reliable? What's their motive?
  • What conclusion does the data actually support?

Success Criteria

□ You identified one specific piece of information you recently accepted.

□ You wrote answers to all four analysis questions and completed the full grid honestly.

Troubleshooting

If you can't identify any biases, you're not digging deep enough. Everyone has biases. Ask, "What would I lose if this were false?" If you couldn't think of questions to ask, start with "Who benefits?" and "What evidence would change my mind?" If you concluded the source is perfectly reliable and has no motive, you're being naive. Everyone has incentives. If your conclusion perfectly matches what you wanted to believe, run the grid again, with more honesty this time.

Building the Habit

The great part about all of this is that you can develop these skills and build up a process that becomes easier to do over time. Once you critically think about a particular subject or a particular process or a particular thing, and you have your structure set up, all there is to do is to wash, rinse, repeat. And it becomes easier to eliminate your biases. You will get to a point where you don't even really start to form them anymore.

And the great part too is also, as you draw conclusions, you can take that through the process again to see if you arrive at the same conclusions or something different.

Integration: How Collection and Analysis Work Together
Collection without analysis leaves you drowning in data. Analysis without collection leaves you reasoning from insufficient evidence. They're two halves of the same process, and they feed each other:

Good collection gives you diverse, credible inputs to analyze.

Good analysis reveals gaps in your collection, showing you what else you need to gather.

Iteration between the two sharpens both: collect, analyze, identify gaps, collect more, refine analysis

This is why critical thinking isn't a one-time event. It's a loop. The more you practice the loop, the faster and more accurate it becomes. Eventually, the questions become reflexive: "Where did this come from?" "What's the counter-argument?" "What evidence would change my mind?"

EXAMINING SACRED BELIEFS

Religious beliefs are often the ones people are most reluctant to examine. From a religious perspective, using the basic skills outlined here can be confronting. You might say, "I'm a devout [insert religion here]. How dare you tell me to question something I've already been taught was true? Why would you ask me to continue testing those beliefs? Doesn't that show a lack of belief or faith?"

I understand that objection. It feels like betrayal when someone suggests you interrogate the foundations you've built your life on. But here's the principle I operate from: truth will always be true, no matter how much I test and question it. If something is actually true, your questions won't destroy it. They'll strengthen your understanding of why it stands.

Not only are we to test our personal beliefs, but our religious ones as well. Rarely do any of us find truth without experiencing it. Through testing and questioning, you're experiencing. Christianity itself tells you to test it out: "Taste and see that the Lord is good" (Psalm 34:8). The invitation is to experience, not just accept. Paul writes in 1 Thessalonians 5:21, "Test everything; hold fast what is good." This isn't permission to doubt. This is a command to verify.

So, to me, not taking my parents' religion as my own "just because" or not falling into a particular religion because it "feels right" was the only path to go. I needed to know why I believed what I believed. Inherited faith and emotional resonance aren't enough to sustain you when that belief gets hard. You need tested conviction.

I always operate on the premise that truth invites questioning and testing. That is the only way you know what is true. Counterfeits fear examination. Truth welcomes it. A faith that collapses under scrutiny wasn't built on anything solid to begin with. Real faith survives the interrogation because it's anchored in reality, not wishful thinking.

This doesn't mean you approach sacred beliefs with arrogance or cynicism (check the pitfalls section for details on that). You approach them with intellectual honesty and humility, willing to follow the evidence wherever it leads, trusting that if God is real and His Word is true, rigorous examination will confirm rather than contradict that reality.

If you're afraid to question, ask yourself why. Is it because you're worried the answers won't hold up? Or is it because you've been taught that questioning equals unfaithfulness? Those are two different problems. The first requires courage to face what you might find. The second requires courage to reject a definition of faith that treats God like He's too fragile to withstand honest inquiry. Faith, real faith, requires evidence. That is largely contrary to what modern-day philosophers will tell you now. Evidence begs to be examined and analyzed.

Test your beliefs. Question your assumptions. If they're true, they'll still be standing when you're done. And if they're not, you'll have saved yourself years of building on a foundation that was never solid in the first place.

PRACTICE PROMPT

- ❖ Write out your own critical thinking checklist. What steps will you actually follow the next time you need to make an important decision?

❖ Make it simple. Make it yours. Then use it.

Success Criteria

☐ Within the recommended timeframe, you took the action described.

Troubleshooting

If your mind resists this exercise, notice the resistance itself. What belief is protecting you from clarity? Write that down first. Then try again.

WISDOM TYPES AND SOURCES

There are different sorts of wisdom, and they're not morally equal. Human wisdom is practical, street-smart, and useful; demonic or deceptive wisdom dresses itself as cleverness and destroys; godly wisdom is pure, peaceable, gentle, full of mercy and good fruit, without hypocrisy.

The Bible tells us that the wisdom from above has a character and a taste; you can test it by its fruit. Godly wisdom doesn't show up on the cheap; you seek it. It's not random insight that lands by accident; it's the product of humility, Scripture-soaked reflection, and hard practice.

If you sit in your own head in a bubble and never test your view with others or with facts, you won't get wisdom. Wisdom demands you move outward: listen, observe, and be corrected.

James describes wisdom from above: pure, peaceable, gentle, open to reason, full of mercy and good fruits, impartial, and sincere. That description isn't a checklist to be admired from a distance; it's a profile of someone who thinks, speaks, and acts in a way that points to God. When you read James 3:17, you see that heavenly wisdom isn't rough, argumentative cleverness. It's a moral, relational, practical knowing that shows up as steadiness and fruit in real life.

Wisdom training operates at the evaluation step of the framework. Once you've perceived accurately and comprehended clearly, you need to judge whether your conclusions are sound. Human reasoning alone has limits. Wisdom is the divine element that elevates evaluation beyond logic and evidence, adding discernment that comes from God. This section shows you how to integrate spiritual wisdom into your decision-making process, ensuring your evaluations aren't just intellectually sound but spiritually grounded.

Three Types of Wisdom in the Same Situation

The scenario is this: A friend asks for financial advice.

Your friend is considering a risky investment opportunity with high potential return but also high potential loss. They ask what you think.

Human wisdom says, "Look at the track record. Calculate the risk. Diversify your portfolio. Don't invest more than you can afford to lose." This is practical, street-smart, and useful. It draws on experience and data. It's good advice as far as it goes, but it lacks moral and relational depth.

Demonic/Deceptive wisdom says, "You deserve this. Everyone else is getting rich. Why shouldn't you? If you don't take this risk, you'll regret it forever. Besides, if it goes bad, you can always declare bankruptcy." This sounds clever and empowering, but it's destructive. It appeals to greed, comparison, and fear. It prioritizes gain over integrity and ignores consequences.

Godly wisdom says, "Let's pray about this first. Have you sought counsel from others who know finances and know your situation? What does Scripture say about debt, stewardship, and contentment? If this goes wrong, how will it affect your family and your ability to serve? Is this driven by need, greed, or genuine opportunity? Let's make sure your peace and your relationships aren't sacrificed for potential gain."

Seemingly Wise

All three responses sound wise on the surface. Only one is rooted in humility, seeks God's direction, prioritizes relationships, and weighs long-term consequences with moral clarity. That's the difference. Godly wisdom doesn't just calculate. It discerns.

You taught yourself to trust your gut long before you ever learned to test a premise; that's physical intuition. It's fast and leans on pattern recognition, and it's useful . . . until it isn't. The Bible and teaching resources urge us to test inner promptings against discernment and Scripture because what feels right can be wrong. Intuition can be a tool, but it's not the whole toolbox for spiritual judgment; wisdom as James describes it moves beyond private hunch into moral clarity that can be examined and trusted.

God's Promise

Here's the promise and the method rolled together: if you lack wisdom, ask God for it. He gives generously to those who ask without doubting. That's the radical simplicity of James 1:5. You don't hustle more experience until God gives you sight; you ask, and while you should still work and learn, you don't neglect the spiritual channel that actually supplies the gift.

That means prayer with expectancy and a posture that says, "I want this, I need this, and I believe you'll give it." Ask plainly and with faith, then watch for how God begins to shape your thinking and decisions.

A Caution

Don't misunderstand the prayer as magic without preparation. Scripture places a foundation under the request: fear of the Lord is the beginning of wisdom; that reverent orientation to God is the entry point where divine insight can land and stick. If you don't respect the source, you'll mistake your own cleverness for God's voice. Reverence and humility tune you to receive rather than project. That fear isn't terror; it's awe that reorders your priorities and opens you to instruction rather than stubborn self-sufficiency.

There are practical prerequisites that make you a soil befitting that gift. The Scriptures and topical guides point to things that prepare the heart:

- consistent immersion in God's Word
- steady prayer that includes listening not just talking
- keeping wise company so you're shaped by people who reflect godly insight
- cultivating inner purity and sincerity so hypocrisy doesn't block what's given

In short, you don't build a wisdom-filled life by accident;

you prepare the environment in which wisdom can be given and received. Surround yourself with people who model heavenly wisdom and stop parking in circles that feed cynicism or constant doubt.

Then there are daily disciplines that actually sharpen the sense:

- Read Scripture slowly and meditatively, not just to check a box but to let the Word reframe how you perceive choices.

- Journal prayers and responses so you can track nudges and outcomes and learn to distinguish genuine leading from wishful thinking.

- Practice listening in prayer: speak less, sit longer, and learn to notice the "still, small" movement and the practical confirmations that follow your asking.

- Test what you think you heard with Scripture, wise counsel, and small experiments before you act broadly. Those habits turn asking into discerned receiving, not mystical guessing.

- Stitch worship and community to the whole process.

Many devotional resources and study guides underscore that prayerful community and deliberate habits, a rhythm of asking, listening, testing, and obeying are how wisdom gets practical legs. When you live in that loop, you'll begin to notice two things: your decisions become calmer and clearer, and your intuition gets upgraded by a pattern of confirmations that point back to a divine record, not just personal pattern-matching.

Wisdom still uses your experience but isn't limited to it; it can draw on what's given by God beyond your history, and that's what makes it both supernatural and usable in daily life.

So here's the short, blunt play:

- Ask God for wisdom (and do it confidently).
- Clean up the soil (fear God, study Scripture, keep wise company, cultivate sincerity).

- Build listening habits (prayer, journaling, small tests).
- And let your physical intuition be corrected and strengthened by what you are given.

The result is having judgment that looks less like luck and more like trained sight and having wisdom that produces fruit, heals relationships, and steadies your path when life heats up.

Wisdom provides direction, but direction alone won't build the capacity to follow it. You need practices—repeatable, daily disciplines—that strengthen your attention, sharpen your discernment, and create the mental infrastructure for you to have sound judgment. These aren't optional add-ons. They're the foundation on which everything else rests.

PRACTICE PROMPT

❖ Pick one decision you need to make this week. Write down: "God, I need wisdom about [specific situation]. Show me what to do."

❖ Track these daily for one week:
  - **Scripture**—What verses speak to this?
  - **Counsel**—What did wise people say?
  - **Confirmation**—What patterns or peace showed up?

❖ At week's end, review for clear direction.

Success Criteria

☐ You identified one specific decision.
☐ You wrote your request to God.
☐ You tracked Scripture/counsel/confirmation daily for seven days.
☐ You consulted two people before deciding.

Troubleshooting

If no Scripture spoke to it, try reading Proverbs with your question in mind. If you didn't ask anyone, start with one trusted person. If nothing's clear after seven days, extend tracking another week.

If your two consultants disagreed, ask a third or wait longer.

HOW MEDITATION HELPS

I used to say meditation was for suckers, but that was until I got good at it. The truth is, it's where the work begins because it teaches you to sit in a moment without running. I can't overstate how important it is to think about what you're thinking about. Five seconds of pause is where lives get saved.

Start small: ten minutes a day, count breaths, label thoughts with simple categories (such as planning, fear, memory, impulse), and bring your focus back without drama. Build to fifteen, then twenty. The point isn't to empty your mind like a TV ad for wellness; it's to strengthen attention so when your heart wants to sprint, your head can put a logical leash on it and ask, "Okay, now what's actually running this?"

Meditation supports the entire framework by training the attention muscle that makes every other step possible. You can't perceive accurately if your mind is scattered. You can't comprehend deeply if you're distracted. You can't evaluate soundly if you're reactive. And you can't decide confidently if you lack mental discipline. Meditation builds the foundational capacity for sustained focus and emotional regulation that allows the framework to function.

This section teaches you how to train your mind to stay present, notice what's happening internally, and return to center when pulled off course.

During the Process of Meditation

You set a timer for ten minutes. You sit. You start counting breaths. Inhale (one), exhale (one), inhale (two), exhale (two) . . . By breath three, your mind has already wandered. It might look like this:

Thought: "I need to email that client. Wait, did I send that invoice? I should check my calendar . . ." You notice. **You label it: planning.** You return to the breath. No judgment. Just return.

Thought: "What if that presentation goes badly? What if they don't like it? What if I forget what to say?" You notice. **Label: fear.** Return to the breath.

Thought: "Remember that time at the UPS job when . . ." You

102

notice. **Label: memory.** Return.

Thought: "I should check my phone. This is boring. I could be doing something productive." **Label: impulse.** Return.

This happens dozens of times in ten minutes. That's not failure; that's the work. Each time you notice a thought, label it, and return to the breath, you're building the muscle. You're training your mind to recognize when it's been hijacked and to come back to center.

After weeks of this, something shifts.

The Shift

In conversations, you notice when anger is rising before it takes over. In decisions, you catch assumptions before they become conclusions. In reactions, you find a pause where there used to be only a reflex.

That's the payoff.

Meditation doesn't make you calm all the time. It makes you aware of when you're not calm, and it gives you the option to choose your response instead of defaulting to reaction.

Meditation builds the attention muscle, the ability to notice what's happening in your mind and return to base. But attention alone isn't enough.

You also need the skill to evaluate what you're noticing. You need to separate signal from noise, truth from manipulation, solid reasoning from clever rhetoric. That's where critical thinking becomes operational. If meditation is the pause button, critical thinking is the diagnostic tool you use during the pause.

PRACTICE PROMPT

- ❖ Set a timer for ten minutes. Sit. Count breaths. When thoughts come, label them (planning, fear, memory, impulse), and return to the breath.

- ❖ Afterward, write down which category showed up most. What does that tell you about what's running in the background of your mind?

Success Criteria

◻ You completed a ten-minute meditation session, labeling thoughts as they appeared.
◻ You identified which category showed up most.
◻ You wrote what this reveals about your mental background noise.
◻ You repeated this for three consecutive days.

Troubleshooting

If you couldn't sit for ten minutes, start with five. If you forgot to label thoughts, don't worry, as that's normal at first. Just notice and label when you remember.

If you can't identify a dominant category, then all categories are running equally, which means your mind is scattered. Keep practicing.

If nothing showed up, you fell asleep or zoned out. Try meditating at a different time of day when you're more alert.

HATCHET MOVES

You can build the best critical thinking habits in the world, practice meditation daily, develop sophisticated frameworks for decision-making, and still get nowhere if your mental environment is poisoned. Think of it this way: you wouldn't train for a marathon while breathing coal smoke. The strongest lungs can't compensate for toxic air. The same principle applies to your mind.

The solution isn't subtle or gradual. It requires what I call "hatchet moves," deliberate, surgical cuts that remove toxicity at the source. These aren't suggestions or mild adjustments. They're structural changes that physically alter your environment and daily patterns.

Habitual negativity and enabling sin are cognitive static. They trash your thinking over time.

You need radical, practical moves.

The Framework

Identify a source of daily toxicity. Don't say vague categories, but specific, nameable things: a news feed, a friendship, or a habit.

Then, enact hard rules, time limits, or accountability structures. Move an app behind a password. Delay exposure to it that day until you've read something that challenges you. Delete entirely if necessary.

Cutting as the only action creates a void, and voids get filled with whatever's closest. So replace what you remove with something that builds rather than drains:

- Five minutes of breathwork
- A page of demanding reading
- One small gratitude note written

You change the environment and the inputs because you can't out-think bad wiring.

Reducing Toxicity Sources

Toxicity Source #1 is doom-scrolling the news.

Here is the pattern: You wake up, grab your phone, and scroll through headlines that are designed to trigger fear, outrage, or anxiety. By 8:00 AM, you're mentally exhausted and your worldview is darker than it was when you went to sleep.

This is a hatchet move: Have a hard rule, such as no news before 10:00 AM. Set your phone to grayscale mode until then.

Make a structural change: Delete news apps. Bookmark two high-quality long-form sources, and check them once daily at a scheduled time.

Fill the Void: Your morning routine becomes ten minutes of meditation, fifteen minutes of Scripture or a challenging book, and then the news if needed.

Toxicity Source #2 is a draining friendship.

Here is the pattern: You have a friend who only calls to complain, never to celebrate. Every conversation leaves you exhausted. They demand emotional labor but offer nothing in return.

This is a hatchet move: Have a hard rule to limit contact to once per month. Don't answer every call immediately.

Accountability: Tell one trusted person: "I'm setting boundaries with this friendship. Check on me in thirty days."

Fill the Void: Invest that time in a reciprocal friendship, someone who gives and receives mutually.

Harder Cuts: Toxicity That Feels Good

The two examples above are relatively straightforward because the toxicity is obvious. You feel worse after engaging. But what about sources that give you a hit of pleasure while slowly poisoning your mind? These are the ones most people protect because cutting them feels like punishment rather than liberation. Social media isn't just scrolling. It's the dopamine cycle of validation. You know the comparison trap is wrecking you, but you still check how many likes you got. The "fun" friend who's a bad influence—you know they're pulling you toward sin, but they're entertaining, and you don't want to seem uptight. The show that normalizes sexual immorality or glorifies violence—you binge it anyway because it's well-made and everyone's talking about it. The work environment that's toxic but pays well—you tell yourself you'll leave eventually while your soul gets ground down daily.

These sources are harder to cut because they don't announce themselves as poison. They feel like reward. That's precisely why they're more dangerous. If toxicity that feels bad can wreck your thinking, toxicity that feels good will do it faster and deeper because you'll defend it, rationalize it, and refuse to name it.

The hatchet move is the same: name it, set a hard boundary, replace it. But expect more resistance. Your flesh will fight you on these because it's getting something out of the exchange. That resistance is proof you need to cut.

The principle is simple: you cannot out-think a toxic environment. If your inputs are poisoned, your outputs will be, too. Cut the source. Replace it with something that builds rather than drains. Protect the infrastructure.

PRACTICE PROMPT

Name two specific sources of toxicity. Don't talk in vague terms. Be direct. Use actual names. Then for each one, write one structural change you'll make this week. Delete the app? Unfollow? Set a timer? Write it down, then do it this week.

Success Criteria

☐ You identified two specific toxic sources by name.
☐ You wrote one structural change for each.
☐ You made both changes this week and filled each void with a building practice.

Troubleshooting

If you can't name specific sources, you're being too general. Look at what drains you daily.

If you named them but didn't make the changes, you're choosing toxicity over growth. Start with one source instead of two.

If you made the changes but didn't fill the void, you'll relapse. Nature abhors a vacuum.

If you swapped one news app for another, you didn't cut toxicity; you relocated it.

COMMON PITFALLS

Training a sound mind is not complicated, but it's easy to derail if you don't know where people typically fail. These are the traps that look like progress but actually keep you stuck. Learn to recognize them. Avoid them. Move forward.

Pitfall 1: Analysis Paralysis

The trap is over-evaluating to the point of never deciding. You use critical thinking as an excuse to avoid action.

You tell yourself you need more data, more clarity, more time. But what you really need is the courage to decide. The Perceive and Comprehend components are meant to sharpen judgment, not stall movement. At some point, you have enough information. The problem isn't data; it's fear.

Say you're deciding between job offers. You research both companies. You read every review, talk to fifteen employees, and analyze salary projections, commute times, and office culture. Six weeks later, you're still "gathering information" while both offers expire. You weren't being thorough. You were avoiding commitment.

The fix is to set decision deadlines. Act even if you only have 80% certainty. Perfect information doesn't exist. A sound mind makes good decisions with incomplete data and adjusts if needed. Proverbs 27:1 warns us not to procrastinate.

"Boast not thyself of tomorrow; for thou knowest not what a day may bring forth" (Proverbs 27:1).

Delayed obedience is disobedience. Decide.

Pitfall 2: False Intellectualism

The trap is confusing information consumption with wisdom. You read ten books but never apply one insight.

This is the person who's "always learning" but never changing. They can quote philosophers, recite studies, and explain cognitive biases, but their life doesn't reflect any of it. They're intellectual tourists, visiting ideas but never moving in. They've mastered perception and comprehension but refuse to act.

For example, you've read three books on time management, listened to five podcasts on productivity, and bookmarked twenty articles on focus. Yet you still procrastinate, miss deadlines, and spend hours scrolling. Knowledge without application is entertainment, not transformation.

The fix is the Act component because it forces application. After learning something, implement it within twenty-four hours.

One concept. One action. Repeat.

James 1:22 is clear:

"Be ye doers of the word and not hearers only, deceiving your own selves" (James 1:22).

Stop collecting information. Start living it.

Pitfall 3: Spiritual Bypassing

The trap is using "I'll pray about it" to avoid critical thinking. You expect divine revelation while refusing to use God-given reasoning.

This is lazy faith disguised as humility. God gave you a mind.

Use it. Prayer isn't a substitute for moving through the decision framework; it's the foundation that strengthens every step. You still need to perceive accurately, comprehend deeply, evaluate soundly, and act decisively.

For example, you're offered a business opportunity that sounds too good to be true. The numbers are vague, the promises are grand, and red flags are everywhere. Instead of evaluating the evidence, you say, "I'll pray about it" and hope God sends a sign. Two weeks later, you invest, lose money, and blame "God's will." That wasn't faith. That was abdication.

The fix is knowing that prayer doesn't replace the framework; it supports it. Pray for wisdom, then use your mind.

Perception: What are the observable facts?

Comprehension: What do these facts mean?

Evaluation: What's the evidence this is sound?

Decision: What does wisdom counsel?

Act: Execute with confidence.

Proverbs 2:6 promises:

"For the Lord giveth wisdom: out of his mouth cometh knowledge and understanding" (Proverbs 2:6).

He expects you to use it.

Pitfall 4: Perception Distortion

The trap is seeing what you want to see instead of what's actually there. Your biases corrupt the data before you even comprehend it.

Most people don't observe; they project. They filter every situation through fear, desire, or expectation. When perception is compromised, every step thereafter fails. You can't comprehend accurately if you're working with distorted data.

For example, your spouse seems distant lately. Your perception says, "They're pulling away. They don't love me anymore." You spiral into anxiety, withdraw emotionally, and create the very distance you feared. The reality you missed is that they were stressed about work and needed space to process. Your distorted perception wrecked what you were trying to protect.

The fix is to separate facts from interpretation. Before reacting, pause and write down only observable data. What did they actually say? What did they actually do? Strip away your assumptions, fears, and hopes. A sound mind observes reality as it is, not as it fears it might be. Only after accurate perception can you move to sound comprehension.

Pitfall 5: Pride in Understanding

The trap is the way your sharp mind makes you insufferable. You correct everyone, dismiss opposing views without listening, and treat disagreement as ignorance.

You've trained your perception and comprehension. You see patterns others miss. You understand complexity. And now you're arrogant. You use your trained mind to dominate conversations rather than serve people. This isn't wisdom; it's pride. And pride makes you stupid.

For example, you're in a meeting. Someone shares an idea you think is flawed. Instead of asking clarifying questions or exploring their reasoning, you immediately explain why they're wrong, condescendingly. The conversation shuts down. You won the argument, but you lost influence. And you missed the chance to learn something you didn't see.

The fix is to be patient and humble.

A sound mind serves; it doesn't dominate. 1 Corinthians 8:1 warns, "Knowledge puffeth up, but charity edifieth." Listen more than you speak. Ask questions before you explain. Teach with patience, not contempt. The goal of training your mind isn't to prove you're smarter; it's to make better decisions and help others do the same.

Pitfall 6: Isolation from Counsel

The trap is thinking you don't need input from others. A sound mind operating alone becomes an echo chamber.

You've trained your perception, sharpened your comprehension, and refined your evaluation. So why do you need other people's opinions? Because you're still finite. Your blind spots are real, and you can't see them alone. A sound mind that refuses counsel is a fortress with no windows.

For example, you're planning a major career move. You've run through the entire framework: perceived the facts, comprehended the implications, evaluated the options, decided on the path. But you haven't talked to anyone—not your spouse, not a mentor, not a trusted friend. You launch the plan, and it fails spectacularly because of something obvious to everyone else but invisible to you. Proverbs 15:22 says this:

"Without counsel purposes are disappointed: but in the multitude of counselors they are established"
(Proverbs 15:22).

The fix is to seek input from people you trust and respect, not people who just agree with you but people who will challenge your thinking and expose your blind spots. Submit major decisions to counsel. Listen. Adjust. Then decide. A sound mind doesn't fear other perspectives; it seeks them.

Pitfall 7: Reactive Impulsivity

The trap is skipping the entire framework and going straight from perception to action. That is the opposite of analysis paralysis.

This is the person who acts so fast they skip comprehension, evaluation, and decision altogether. They perceive a situation and immediately react. No pause. No thought. Just reflex. You see something and move before you understand what you're looking at. Speed feels like decisiveness, but it's just recklessness.

For example,

you read a headline that angers you. Within seconds, you share it on social media with a heated caption, tag three people, and fire off your opinion. Two hours later, you read the actual article and realize the headline was misleading. The story is more nuanced than you thought. But you've already created conflict, damaged your credibility, and can't unsend what you sent. You perceived accurately but moved too fast to comprehend.

The fix is to build in a mandatory pause between perception and action. When you feel the urge to react immediately, that's your signal to slow down. Count to ten. Write out what you observed before you respond. Ask yourself: "Do I understand this fully?" Proverbs 29:20 warns us:

"Seest thou a man that is hasty in his words? There is

more hope of a fool than of him" (Proverbs 29:20).

A sound mind creates space between stimulus and response. Speed without thought is not decisiveness; it's impulsivity.

Pitfall 8: Confirmation Bias

The trap is selectively gathering and accepting only evidence that confirms what you already believe.

This is different from perception distortion. You're not misinterpreting what you see; you're refusing to look at half of what's there. You only ask people who will agree with you. You only read sources that support your view. You dismiss challenges as ignorance. You're not seeking truth; you're seeking validation. And validation masquerading as investigation will wreck you.

For example, you believe your business idea is brilliant. You pitch it only to supportive friends. When experienced entrepreneurs raise concerns, you write them off as "stuck in old thinking" or "risk-averse." You read three articles that validate your approach and ignore five that challenge it. You launch. It fails. The warnings were there. You just refused to see them because they threatened what you wanted to believe.

The fix is to actively seek disconfirming evidence. Before you decide, ask, "What would prove me wrong? Who disagrees with me and why?" Read the strongest arguments against your position. Talk to people who see it differently. If you can't steelman the opposing view (the opposite of "strawman," this means to articulate the strongest and most compelling form of the argument against you), you don't yet understand the issue well enough to decide.

"He that is first in his own cause seemeth just; but

his neighbor cometh and searcheth him" (Proverbs 18:17).

A sound mind doesn't fear contradiction; it pursues it.

Pitfall 9: Intellectual Cowardice

The trap is that you have the capacity for sound thinking but refuse to use it when it might create tension or cost you something.

Your mind works fine. You perceive accurately, comprehend deeply, evaluate soundly. But when speaking the truth would cause conflict, threaten your position, or make you unpopular, you stay silent. You see the problem but pretend you don't. You have the analysis but lack the courage to deploy it. Knowledge without courage is cowardice dressed in humility.

For example, you're in a leadership meeting. The proposed strategy has obvious flaws you can see clearly. Everyone else seems supportive. Rather than voice concerns and risk being "the difficult one," you stay silent and let the group proceed. The strategy fails predictably six months later. You had the insight. You chose silence over service. That's not wisdom; that's fear.

The fix is to pair a sound mind with a courageous heart. If you see something, say something, even when it's uncomfortable. Your responsibility isn't to be liked; it's to be truthful. Speak with respect, but speak.

"If thou forbear to deliver them that are drawn unto death . . . Doth not he that pondereth the heart consider it?" (Proverbs 24:11–12).

Truth unspoken is truth abandoned. Train your courage alongside your mind. Start small: speak one uncomfortable truth this week. Then another. Build the muscle.

PRACTICE PROMPT

❖ Answer these nine questions honestly. Write your answers down. Don't skip any. Don't soften them. If you lie here, you're lying to yourself.
   - Am I using evaluation as an excuse to avoid deciding? (Analysis Paralysis)
   - Am I consuming information without acting on it? (False Intellectualism)
   - Am I praying instead of thinking, or thinking without praying? (Spiritual Bypassing)
   - Am I perceiving reality or projecting my fears onto it? (Perception Distortion)
   - Am I using my trained mind to serve others, or prove myself? (Pride)
   - When did I last seek counsel from someone I respect?

(Isolation)

- Do I react before I fully understand what I'm responding to? (Reactive Impulsivity)
- Am I only seeking evidence that confirms what I already believe? (Confirmation Bias)
- Do I stay silent when my sound thinking might create conflict? (Intellectual Cowardice)

❖ After answering, pick the pitfall you fall into most often. Write down one specific example from the last two weeks. Then commit to one corrective action this week.

Success Criteria

☐ You answered all nine questions honestly.
☐ You identified your dominant pitfall.
☐ You wrote down a recent, specific example.
☐ You chose one corrective action from the corresponding "Fix" section and implemented it within seven days.

Troubleshooting

If no pitfall resonates, you likely have blind spots these nine don't capture. Ask someone close to you which one they see in you most often. External perspective reveals what self-assessment can't.

If you identified the pitfall but didn't take corrective action, know that awareness without movement is just informed stagnation.

If the pitfall showed up again even after implementing the fix, that's okay because it's normal. Patterns don't break in a week. The goal is to catch it faster each time.

OTHERS' FAULTY ARGUMENTS

You've built your framework. You've identified your personal pitfalls. Now you need to recognize when someone else's argument is broken.

This isn't about winning debates or embarrassing people. It's about discernment. You need to separate sound reasoning from manipulation, truth from cleverly disguised error, wisdom from smooth-talking nonsense.

Bad arguments are everywhere: news media, social media, marketing, politics, workplace conversations, even church discussions. Most people don't lie outright—they just reason poorly. And if you can't spot faulty reasoning, you'll believe things that aren't true and make decisions based on arguments that don't hold up. This verse warns us:

"The simple believes everything, but the prudent gives thought to his steps" (Proverbs 14:15).

A sound mind doesn't accept arguments just because they seem good at first blush. It evaluates them.

Here are the most common reasoning errors you'll encounter. Learn to recognize them. Once you see them, you can't unsee them.

Ad Hominem: Attacking the Person Not the Argument

It looks like attacking person and not their premise. Instead of addressing what someone said, you attack their character, credentials, or motives. "Of course you support that policy— you're biased." This dodges the actual argument by discrediting the person making it.

For example, your coworker proposes a budget restructure.

Instead of evaluating the proposal, someone says, "Well, he's the one who screwed up last quarter's report, so why should we listen to him now?"

The proposal might be excellent, but the group dismisses it without examination because they attacked the person.

It works because it's easier to dismiss a person than engage an idea. Plus, if others already distrust that person, the attack feels satisfying. But truth doesn't depend on who speaks it.

Here's a Biblical counter: Even Balaam's donkey spoke truth (Numbers 22:28–30). God can use anyone. Proverbs 18:17 warns:

"The one who states his case first seems right, until the other comes and examines him" (Proverbs 15:17).

Examine the argument itself, not just who's making it.

Respond when someone attacks character instead of ideas by asking, "What specifically is wrong with the argument itself?" Force the conversation back to substance. If the person's character genuinely matters (e.g., a pattern of deception), address that separately—but still evaluate the argument on its merits.

Strawman: Misrepresenting to Win

What it looks like: Someone distorts your position into something weaker or more extreme, then attacks that distorted version instead of what you actually said. They're fighting a "straw man" instead of your real argument.

For example, you suggest your church should be more intentional about welcoming visitors. Someone responds, "So you think we should compromise biblical truth to make unbelievers comfortable?" That's not what you said. They twisted "intentional welcoming" into "compromise truth," then attacked the twisted version.

It works because the distorted argument is easier to defeat. And if done skillfully, listeners might not notice the switch. They just hear the person "winning" the argument against something you never said.

Here's a Biblical counter: The Pharisees constantly did this to Jesus. They twisted His words about the temple (John 2:19–21) and His identity (John 10:33). Jesus always brought the conversation back to what He actually said, not their distortion.

Respond by immediately clarifying, "That's not what I said. Let me restate my actual position." Then force them to address your real argument, not their caricature of it.

False Dilemma: Limiting the Options

It looks like presenting only two options when more exist. "Either you support this policy completely, or you don't care about people." This forces you into an artificial choice.

For example, your church is discussing worship style. Someone says, "Either we stick with traditional hymns, or we abandon biblical worship entirely." That's absurd. There are dozens of worship approaches that are both contemporary and biblical. The false dichotomy tries to eliminate nuanced thinking.

It works because it simplifies complex issues, which feels decisive and strong. And if one option is clearly unacceptable, the other "wins" by default—even if better alternatives exist.

Here's a Biblical counter: When Satan tempted Jesus to throw himself from the temple (Matthew 4:5–7), he implied only two options: trust God (jump) or doubt him (don't jump). Jesus rejected the false dichotomy entirely. Refusing to test God wasn't doubt; it was wisdom.

Respond by asking, "What are we not considering?" or "Are those really the only two options?" Expand the conversation beyond the artificial binary setup.

Appeal to Authority: Because the Expert Said So

It looks like accepting something as true simply because an authority figure said it, without evaluating the claim itself. "Doctor Smith says this, so it must be right." Authority figures can be wrong.

For example, someone quotes a celebrity pastor to settle a theological debate. "Pastor Johnson preaches at a megachurch, so his interpretation must be correct." The size of the person's platform doesn't guarantee accuracy. The argument needs to stand on Scripture and reason, not celebrity.

It works because we trust authorities, often rightfully so. Experts usually know more than laypeople. But expertise in one area doesn't equal infallibility, and even experts can be biased, mistaken, or corrupted. Here's a Biblical counter to that logical fallacy. In Galatians 1:8, Paul is as direct as you can get:

"Even if we or an angel from heaven should preach to you a gospel contrary to the one we preached to you, let him be accursed" (Galatians 1:8).

Paul says even apostles and angels can be wrong. Authority doesn't override truth. The Bereans checked Paul's teaching against Scripture daily (Acts 17:11)—they didn't just accept it because Paul said it.

Respond by asking, "What's the evidence for that claim?" or "Can we evaluate the reasoning independent of who's saying it?" Respect expertise, but verify the argument.

Slippery Slope: One Thing Leading to Everything

It looks like claiming that one action will inevitably lead to extreme, undesirable outcomes without showing why the progression is inevitable. "If we allow this small change, soon we'll be in complete chaos."

For example, your church considers adding a second service time. Someone objects: "If we add a second service, soon we'll have three, then four, and before you know it, we'll be a seeker-sensitive megachurch that doesn't preach the gospel anymore." That's a massive leap with no logical connection between steps.

It works because fear of extreme outcomes is powerful. And because bad slopes do exist (addiction, debt), people assume all slopes are slippery. But many aren't. Adding a service time doesn't automatically lead to doctrinal compromise.

Here's a Biblical counter: God's commands often include boundaries precisely because not everything leads to disaster. Paul distinguishes between food offered to idols (which might cause weaker believers to stumble) and food in general (which doesn't). Some slopes are slippery; others aren't. Discernment is required.

Respond by asking: "What evidence do you have that one step inevitably leads to the next?" Make them show the logical connection, not just assert it.

Red Herring: Changing the Subject

It looks like introducing an irrelevant point to distract from the actual issue under discussion. When the argument isn't going well, shift to something else entirely.

For example, your family is discussing whether to take on more debt for a vacation. When you raise financial concerns, someone says, "You just don't value family time together." That's irrelevant. The question isn't about valuing family time — it's about whether this specific expense is wise. They changed the subject to avoid addressing your actual concern.

It works because it derails the conversation and puts you on defense about something else. Now you're defending your commitment to family instead of discussing the budget. The original issue gets buried.

Here's a Biblical counter to that fallacy. When the Pharisees brought the woman caught in adultery to Jesus (John 8:3–11), they were setting a trap. But notice: they made no mention of the man, though adultery requires two people. Jesus redirected to the real issue (their own adultery), then addressed the woman with grace. He didn't let them control the conversation with their selective outrage.

Respond by identifying it immediately: "That's a separate issue. Let's finish discussing [original topic] first, then we can address that if you want." Don't let the conversation drift.

Hasty Generalization: Jumping to Broad Conclusions

It looks like drawing sweeping conclusions from insufficient evidence. "I met two people from that church and they were both judgmental, so the whole church must be full of judgmental people."

For example, your friend tries a diet for one week, loses two pounds, and declares: "This is the answer to everyone's weight problems!" One week, one person, minimal results—yet they've generalized to "everyone." That's hasty.

It works because We love patterns and answers. A small sample feels like enough if it confirms what we want to believe. Plus, our experiences feel representative even when they're not.

Here's a Biblical counter: Proverbs 18: 13 and James 1:19 both address this.

"If one gives an answer before he hears, it is his folly and shame" (Proverbs 18:13). "Let every person be quick to hear, slow to speak" (James 1:19).

Premature conclusions are foolish. Gather sufficient evidence before forming judgments.

Respond by asking, "How many examples are you basing that on?" or "Is that sample size large enough to draw that conclusion?" Push for more evidence before accepting the generalization.

Post Hoc: Confusing Correlation with Causation

It looks like assuming that because one thing happened after another, the first caused the second. "I prayed, then I got the job, so prayer caused the job offer." Maybe. Or maybe you were qualified and the timing was coincidental.

For example, someone starts taking a new supplement and within two weeks feels more energetic. They conclude the supplement works. But they also started sleeping better that week, reduced stress, and ate more vegetables. Which factor caused the improvement? They don't know, but they've assumed it was the supplement because it came first chronologically.

It works because our brains are wired to find causes. When X happens, then Y happens, we instinctively link them. But correlation (things happening together) doesn't prove causation (one causing the other).

Here's a Biblical counter: Scripture warns against false prophets who claim credit for God's work (Deuteronomy 13:1–3). Just because someone prayed and then something happened doesn't mean the prayer caused it—though it might have. Discernment is required. Test the pattern, don't assume it.

Respond by asking, "What else could explain that outcome?" or "Is there evidence that the first thing actually caused the second?" Look for alternative explanations before accepting causation.

Appeal to Emotion: Feelings Over Facts

It looks like manipulating emotions instead of making a logical argument. "How can you not support this cause? Think of the children!" The argument depends on emotional reaction, not reason.

For example, a charity shows heartbreaking images of suffering and asks for donations. The need might be real, but they're not telling you how the money will be used, what percentage goes to overhead, or whether their programs actually work. They're relying on your emotional response to bypass rational evaluation. **It works because** emotions are powerful and fast. Logic is slow and requires effort. If someone can trigger strong feelings (guilt, fear, pity, anger), they can often get you to act without thinking.

Here's a Biblical counter: Jesus often moved people emotionally, but never by manipulation. His emotions were genuine, and his arguments were sound.

"There is a way that seems right to a man, but its end is the way to death" (Proverbs 14:12).

What feels right isn't always true.

Respond by acknowledging the emotion without letting it dictate your conclusion: "Yes, that's heartbreaking. Now let's evaluate whether this specific solution actually addresses the problem." Feel deeply, think clearly.

Bandwagon: Everyone Believes It

It looks like claiming something is true or right because many people believe it. "Everyone's doing it, so it must be okay." Popularity doesn't equal truth.

For example, a financial advisor pitches you on cryptocurrency because "everyone's getting into it." That's not an argument for whether it's a sound investment for your situation. Millions of people can be wrong simultaneously (see: housing bubble, dot-com crash).

It works because we're social creatures. We trust consensus and fear being left out. If everyone else believes something, it feels safe to believe it too. Contrarians risk looking foolish.

Here's a Biblical counter: Jesus warned about the broad path many follow versus the narrow path few find (Matthew 7:13–14). Popularity has never been God's measure of truth. Noah's generation thought he was insane. Elijah stood alone against 450 prophets of Baal. The crowd chose Barabbas over Jesus. Truth isn't democratic.

Respond by asking, "What's the evidence, independent of how many people believe it?" Force the argument to stand on its own merits, not on popularity.

PRACTICE PROMPT

❖ Consume one piece of media this week—a news article, opinion piece, social media thread, or advertisement.

❖ Identify at least three fallacies being used. For each one:
  • Name the fallacy.
  • Quote or describe the specific statement.

- Explain why it's fallacious.
- Rewrite the argument without the fallacy (what a sound version would look like).

Success Criteria

☐ You identified three fallacies with specific examples.
☐ You explained why each was fallacious.
☐ You rewrote at least one argument soundly.

Troubleshooting

If you can't find fallacies, you're either consuming exceptionally rigorous content (rare) or not recognizing them yet (common). Try political commentary, social media debates, or advertising—one you learn to spot them, you will see that fallacies are everywhere. If you found fallacies but can't explain why they're wrong, review the descriptions above, and practice with simpler examples first.

HOW THE ARENAS CONNECT

A sound mind doesn't float above life like an ivory tower. It's the engine that trains the heart, supports the body, and orients the soul. The mind teaches the heart to name feelings and use them as data. The mind helps plan and sustain physical routines that strengthen stamina and self-control, and the body in turn feeds cognitive clarity. The soul provides the moral horizon so the mind can aim at flourishing rather than merely being efficient.

Together, they form a loop: clearer thinking yields calmer emotions, which support healthier bodies and deeper spiritual practices, which then reinforce clearer thinking.

Mind → Heart: Training Emotional Regulation

Your mind is the personal trainer for your heart. When an emotion arises, the mind does the following:

- **Names it accurately:** "I'm feeling anxious" instead of "Something's wrong."
- **Creates the pause:** Meditation builds the gap between feeling and reaction.

- **Provides reframes:** "This anxiety shows I care. How can I prepare instead of panic?"
- **Tests emotional narratives:** "Is this fear based on evidence or assumption?"

Without a sound mind, the heart runs the show. With a sound mind, the heart provides valuable data that the mind can evaluate and direct.

Mind → Body: Planning and Sustaining Physical Discipline

The mind creates the infrastructure for physical consistency:

- **The mind plans training, such as** scheduling workouts like non-negotiable meetings.
- **It maintains discipline,** showing up even when motivation is low.
- **The mind interprets pain signals:** "Is this productive discomfort or injury?"
- **It creates supportive environments, such as** prepping meals, removing junk food, laying out gym clothes.

Body → Mind: Physical Feedback Loop

The body reciprocates:

Exercise boosts cognitive clarity: BDNF (brain-derived neurotrophic factor) from training improves memory and focus

Sleep sharpens judgment: Rest consolidates learning and improves decision-making

Nutrition affects thinking: Blood sugar crashes will cloud your perception.

Mind → Soul: Creating Space for Discernment

The mind prepares the ground for spiritual formation:

Creates contemplation space: Meditation and stillness make room to hear God.

Tests spiritual impressions: "Does this align with Scripture? What do wise counselors say?"

Discerns wisdom from intuition: Distinguishes God's voice from personal preference.

Translates insight to service: Turns spiritual clarity into practical action.

Soul → Mind: Providing Moral Direction

The soul keeps the mind aimed at what matters.**Supplies purpose:** "Why am I thinking about this? What's the goal?"

Guards against clever destruction: Prevents using intelligence for manipulation or harm.

Orients toward flourishing: Ensures the mind serves love, not mere efficiency.

The Integration Loop

Here's how it compounds: A sound mind creates the pause to regulate emotion (heart). Regulated emotion supports disciplined training (body). Physical vitality sharpens cognitive clarity (mind). Mental clarity creates space for prayer and discernment (soul). Spiritual formation provides moral purpose (soul). Moral purpose directs the mind toward wisdom and service. The cycle reinforces itself.

Break the loop at any point, and the whole system weakens. Strengthen any point, and the whole system benefits.

Integration is the goal. But goals without schedules remain aspirational. You need structure, daily, weekly, and long-term plays that turn these practices from good ideas into lived habits. Let's build the actual schedule.

PRACTICE PROMPT

❖ Draw a simple diagram with four circles. Label them Heart, Mind, Body, Soul. Draw arrows showing how they connect. Then answer:
  - How does your mind currently train (or fail to train) your heart?
  - How does your body affect your mind? (Sleep? Exercise? Nutrition?)
  - How does your soul provide direction to your mind?
  - Which connection is weakest? (Where does the loop break down?)
  - What one specific thing will strengthen the weakest link this week?

Success Criteria

☐ You drew the four-arena diagram with connecting arrows.
☐ You answered all of the questions with specific examples.
☐ You identified your weakest connection and wrote one concrete action to strengthen it this week.

Troubleshooting

If you're struggling to see how mind trains heart, review the last week: When did emotion drive a decision? That's a moment where mind could have intervened.

If the body-mind connection isn't clear yet, try this experiment: track your mental sharpness for three days alongside sleep quality and exercise. The pattern will reveal itself.

If you're unsure which link is weakest, it's often the one you thought about last or had the hardest time answering. That hesitation oftentimes is the signal.

If strengthening the weak link feels overwhelming, you're thinking too big. Pick something you can do in five minutes daily.

PRACTICE SCHEDULE

The practice prompts throughout this chapter help you understand and test individual concepts. This section is different: it shows you how to integrate all those practices into one sustainable system. You need structure—daily, weekly, and long-term rhythms that turn these practices from good ideas into lived habits.

What follows is a progressive training schedule that sharpens each step of the decision flow: perception, comprehension, evaluation, decision, and action.

Daily Practices

Do these daily: ten to fifteen minutes of stillness, fifteen minutes of deliberate reading from a challenging book or long-form essay, and a micro-journal entry that answers: What belief did I test today and what did I learn? These small daily acts compound. They tune attention, strengthen perception, force evidence tracking, and habituate the practice of testing rather than mindless absorption.

The Daily Minimum

- Morning (First 30 Minutes Awake):
- 10–15 minutes: Meditation/stillness (trains perception)
- 15 minutes: Challenging reading (trains comprehension and evaluation)
- Evening (Before Bed):
- 3–5 minutes: Micro-journal

Micro-Journal Template

Answer these three questions in one or two sentences each:

1. What belief did I test today?
2. What did I learn?
3. What would I do differently?

Example Entry

Belief tested: "I need coffee to function in the morning."

1. What I learned: Skipped coffee today. Felt sluggish for an hour, then normal. Might be habit, not need.
2. Different next time: Try one more day without coffee to test if it's truly needed or just routine.

Why this works: Daily repetition builds the reflex. Morning practices set the tone before life gets noisy. Evening reflection cements learning. The micro-journal keeps the bar low enough that you'll actually do it.

Weekly and Periodic Practices

On a weekly rhythm, do one forty-minute mental debate (twenty minutes per side) and one information audit where you trace the origin of a strongly held belief and look for gaps.

Do one reframing drill where you rewrite a recurring negative thought three different, calmer ways and practice each for several days.

These weekly exercises sharpen evaluation and strengthen decision-making under pressure.

PRACTICE PROMPT

❖ **Mental Debate (40 minutes, once per week):**

- Pick a topic you have a strong opinion on.
- Set a timer for 20 minutes; argue for your position (write it out).
- Set the timer for 20 minutes; argue *against* your position (write it out).
- Rview both: What surprised you? What weakened? What strengthened?

❖ **Information Audit (30 minutes, once per week):**

- Pick one belief you hold strongly.
- Trace its origin: Where did you first encounter this idea?
- Identify sources: Who said it? What's ther credibility? What's their motive?
- Look for gaps: What counter-evidence have you ignored?

❖ **Reframing Drill (15 minutes, once per week):**

- Identify one recurring negative thought
- Write three different reframes (calmer, evidence-based alternatives)
- Practice one reframe for the next 7 days

Monthly Practice

❖ Review and Adjust (sixty minutes, once per month):
- Review daily journal entries: What patterns emerged?
- Review weekly practices: Which ones helped most? Which felt forced?
- Adjust: What one thing will you change next month?

Quarterly Practice

❖ Wisdom Review (ninety minutes, once per quarter):
- List five to ten significant decisions from the past three months.

- Trace outcomes: What worked? What didn't?
- Identify patterns: What decision-making habits served you? Which ones betrayed you?
- Invite critique: Share your review with one trusted person and ask for their perspective

These periodic checks reveal slow drift and keep the system honest.

A NINETY-DAY PROGRESSIVE PLAN

This plan has three phases, each with its own focus.

Phase one (days one through thirty): build attention and intake discipline. Ten minutes daily sitting, daily reading, one weekly debate.

Phase two (days thirty-one through sixty): harden analytic routines and rehearsals. Add the Question Ladder, increase stillness, start a public accountability practice like a weekly short post where you invite correction.

Phase three (days sixty-one to ninety): expose and integrate. Add one weekly paired drill, run a wisdom review, and invite community feedback. Track simple metrics: the number of uninterrupted meditation minutes per week, number of times you paused before responding to something that once would have set you off, and one qualitative note each week about a decision you handled better. Keep the metrics simple and unobtrusive—the point is habit formation, not score-chasing.

Phase one: Days one through thirty (Foundation)

Your goal is to build your attention and clean up your intake.

Daily

10 minutes meditation
15 minutes deliberate reading
3-sentence micro-journal

Weekly

One 40-minute mental debate

Meditation minutes per week (goal: 70+)
Days journaled (goal: 25+)

Phase two: Days thirty-one through sixty (Deepen)

Your goal is to harden analytic routines. **Add this to your daily list:** Increase meditation to fifteen minutes. **Add these to your weekly list:**

- Question Ladder drill (ask "why" or "how" five times on one belief)
- Information audit (trace origin of one strongly held belief)

Public Accountability

Once per week, post one tentative view and invite correction (blog, group chat, trusted community).

Metrics to Track

The number of times you paused before reacting (goal: Note three or more instances per week.)

Phase three: Days sixty-one through ninety (Integrate)

Your goal is to expose thinking to feedback and integrate practices.

Add this to your weekly list:

Paired drill with trusted friend (forty-five minutes, every two weeks): each presents a view, cross-examines, summarizes surprises

Add this to your monthly list:

Do a sixty-minute review: patterns, adjustments, community feedback.

At the end of ninety days, run a full Wisdom Review.

Invite one trusted critic to evaluate your growth.

Metrics to Track

One qualitative note per week: "This is a decision I handled better this week."

Progressive—Each phase builds on the previous.
Realistic—Daily minimums are achievable (30 minutes total).
Measured—Simple metrics track progress without obsession.
Accountable—Community involvement prevents drift.

The ninety-day structure gives you time to build the muscle memory of sound thinking without overwhelming your current capacity. By day ninety, the practices that felt awkward on day one will have become your new default mode of operation.

MARKERS OF PROGRESS

A sound mind doesn't announce itself with fanfare. It shows up in how you handle pressure, how you make decisions, and how others respond to your presence. These markers tell you the training is working. Use them to measure growth and stay accountable.

In Perception

You notice when you're interpreting vs. observing.

You catch yourself mid-assumption and pause: "Wait, is that what happened, or is that what I think happened?" The gap between data and meaning becomes visible.

You catch yourself making assumptions in real time.

Before, you reacted to interpretations without realizing they were interpretations. Now you see the moment it happens and course-correct.

Other people start asking, "How did you notice that?"

Your perception is sharper than most. You see patterns, inconsistencies, and details others miss. Not because you're smarter but because you're trained.

You're less reactive because you're seeing data, not threats. Criticism doesn't spike your heart rate. Conflict doesn't trigger defensiveness. You observe what's happening without immediately personalizing it.

In Comprehension

You can steelman opposing arguments (argue them better than their proponents) and understand positions you disagree with well enough to articulate them fairly and persuasively. This isn't compromise. It's intellectual honesty.

You grasp nuance and context others miss. You see the complexity in situations and are better at resisting oversimplification.

You understand the "why" behind positions, not just the "what."

Complex ideas become accessible when you teach them. You explain clearly and without condescension. People understand not just what you're saying, but why it matters.

You read between the lines in conversations. You hear what people mean, not just what they say. You pick up on subtext, tone, and unspoken concerns.

In Evaluation

You ask, "What's the source?" automatically. Headlines, hot takes, bold claims—you don't accept them at face value anymore. You trace back to the origin and evaluate credibility. You're harder to manipulate; propaganda feels obvious.

Emotional manipulation, loaded language, appeals to fear— you spot them instantly. Not out of cynicism but because you've trained yourself to test claims before accepting them.

You catch logical fallacies in real-time conversations:

- Ad hominem
- Straw man
- Appeal to authority
- False dichotomy

You hear them as they happen and either address them gracefully or note them internally.

Prayer becomes specific, not generic. You're no longer praying vague requests ("Bless me, guide me"). You're asking for specific wisdom on specific decisions. And you're expecting specific answers.

Scripture speaks to current decisions instead of just feeling inspiring. You read a passage and immediately see how it applies to what you're facing today. The Word isn't just encouraging— it's instructive.

You can distinguish God's voice from your own preferences.

You're learning to tell the difference between "what I want" and "what God is saying." This doesn't happen overnight, but the gap narrows with practice.

Fasting creates clarity, not just hunger. When you fast from distractions, you hear better. The noise quiets. The signal strengthens.

In Decision and Action

Decisions that felt murky become clear. You make decisions faster with equal or better outcomes. You're not impulsive, but you're not paralyzed, either. You process quickly, evaluate soundly, and move. The delay between information and action shrinks.

You second-guess yourself less, and you trust your evaluation process. Once the decision is made, you commit. You don't replay it endlessly looking for flaws.

When you're wrong, you adjust quickly without shame.

Mistakes don't crush you. You see them, acknowledge them, correct course, and move forward. No spiraling. No defensiveness. Just recalibration.

People start trusting your judgment. Others notice the consistency of your decisions. They ask your opinion more often. They trust your counsel because your track record speaks.

In Relationships

Fewer arguments are caused by misunderstanding. You clarify before you react. You ask questions before you assume. Conflicts that used to flare up now dissolve because you're watching perception.

People seek your counsel. Friends, family, colleagues—they come to you when they're stuck. Not because you have all the answers, but because you ask the right questions and help them think clearly.

You can hold tension in disagreement without fracturing. You don't need everyone to agree with you to maintain relationship. You can disagree strongly and still respect deeply. Disagreement doesn't equal disrespect.

Your words carry more weight because your thinking is sound. People listen when you speak because your words are measured, precise, and grounded. You don't talk just to fill silence.

In Ministry/Leadership

Your teaching is clearer. Complex ideas become more accessible.

You explain without condescension. People understand not just what you're saying but why it matters.

Your decisions benefit more people. You think beyond yourself. Your judgment accounts for consequences that ripple beyond the immediate. Leadership isn't just about you anymore.

You're less swayed by trends or popularity. Pressure to conform doesn't move you. You evaluate based on truth, not applause. This makes you steady in chaos.

You can lead through complexity without panic. Uncertainty doesn't paralyze you. You navigate ambiguity, make decisions with incomplete data, and adjust as new information arrives.

Others follow you because you're calm.

COMMON OBSTACLES

The Introduction addressed objections from people deciding whether to start. This section is different. These are obstacles that show up when you're already in the work. You've started training your mind. You've seen some progress. Now you're hitting resistance points that slow or stall the process. These aren't character flaws. They're predictable challenges that surface when the initial motivation fades and you start to work those discipline muscles. Here's how to recognize them and work through them.

Obstacle #1: "I'm overwhelmed by information."

What's Happening

You're exposed to more information in one day than previous generations encountered in a lifetime. Without boundaries, you're drowning in noise and can't distinguish signal.

Why This Happens

Algorithms are designed to maximize engagement, not clarity. The fire hose is intentional. Your overwhelm is profitable to someone.

Institute intake windows: Check news/social media only at set times (10 AM, 3 PM, 7 PM)

- ❖ Two-source rule: Don't act on contested claims until two credible, independent sources confirm.

- ❖ Daily quiet hour: One hour per day with zero information input. Walk. Sit. Think.

- ❖ Unsubscribe ruthlessly: Delete apps, unfollow accounts, cancel subscriptions that add noise.

Obstacle #2: "I'm stuck in my biases."

What's Happening

You've become aware of your biases, which is good. Awareness alone doesn't break patterns. You need active practice to challenge them.

Why This Happens

Biases are cognitive shortcuts that saved energy for thousands of years. Your brain defaults to them because they're efficient, not because they're accurate.

How to Address It

Do a weekly Devil's Advocate Drill: Argue against one of your own beliefs for 20 minutes.

- ❖ Invite honest critique: Ask a trusted friend, "Where am I blind? What am I missing?"

- ❖ Seek disconfirming evidence: Actively hunt for the strongest arguments against what you believe.

- ❖ Track changes: Journal when you change your mind. Celebrate it. Make it normal.

Obstacle #3: "Emotions still hijack me."

What's Happening

You understand the theory of emotional regulation, but in the moment, you still react before thinking. It isn't automatic yet.

Why This Happens

Emotional regulation is a skill like any other. It requires repetition. You wouldn't expect to run a marathon after one week of training. Same principle applies here.

How to Address It

Breathe before responding: Inhale four counts, exhale six counts; repeat five times.

- Take a written pause: When emotion spikes, write it down: "I feel [emotion] because [reason]."

- Require a delay: For consequential choices, wait 24 hours before acting.

- Stack micro habits: Practice in low-stakes moments so the skill is available in high-stakes instances.

Obstacle #4: "I'll start when things calm down."

What's Happening

You're waiting for ideal conditions that never arrive. Life stays chaotic, and the waiting becomes permanent procrastination.

Why This Happens

Starting in chaos feels harder than waiting for calm. But calm is a myth. The chaos is the norm.

How to Address It

Start in the chaos: 5 minutes during lunch, 3 minutes before bed

- Lower the bar: One pushup is better than zero. One sentence journaled is better than none.

- Schedule it like a meeting: Put it on the calendar. Treat it as non-negotiable.

  ❖ Recognize the pattern: If you've been waiting for months,
    the conditions aren't coming. Start now.

Obstacle #5: "This is just how I am."

What's Happening

You've adopted a fixed mindset about your capacity. You believe
your thinking patterns are hardwired and unchangeable.

Why This Happens

Fixed mindset feels safer than growth mindset. If you can't
change, you can't fail. But it also means you can't grow.

How to Address It

  ❖ Read one story of radical change: Someone who was worse
    off than you and changed

  ❖ Reframe identity: Stop saying "I am" and start saying "I
    currently do."

  ❖ Track micro-progress: Small wins break the fixed mindset.
    Write them down.

  ❖ Challenge the narrative: Ask "Is this actually true, or is
    this what I've believed for so long I stopped questioning
    it?"

The Pattern

These obstacles are common because they're human. Most people
encounter at least three of the five. The solution in every case
follows the same structure: start smaller, add friction to bad habits,
remove friction from good habits, and invite accountability. None
of this is perfect. All of it is better than staying stuck.

PRACTICE PROMPT

Which obstacle are you facing right now?

  ❖ Write it down honestly.

  ❖ Then choose one solution from that obstacle's list and

implement it this week. Not all of them. Just one. Start small, and build from there.

Success Criteria

☐ You identified an obstacle currently slowing your progress,
☐ You chose one specific solution and tried it.
☐ You noted what happened.

Did it help? Did it reveal something? Keep what works. Adjust what doesn't.

Troubleshooting

If you identified multiple obstacles, pick the one that made you most uncomfortable when reading it—that's probably your primary blocker.

If you picked a solution but didn't try it, the barrier might be too high. Make it smaller. If you tried it, and it didn't help, either give it more time or try a different solution from the list.

If you can't identify any obstacle, ask someone who knows you well which one they see in you. Their answer matters more than yours.

You've built practices for yourself. You've addressed obstacles. You've created structure. But a sound mind isn't just for you. It's for the people who watch you, learn from you, and come after you. Legacy isn't only money or property. It's cognitive tone, decision-making patterns, and the model you pass forward. Teaching others is how the work compounds beyond your own life.

CONCLUSION

A sound mind is a trained capacity to perceive rightly, evaluate humbly, and decide wisely. It anchors emotion, resists manipulation, and compounds into outcomes that matter for you and everyone after you. Its cultivation is plain work: stillness to train attention, ruthless intake rules to keep input honest, analytic drills to test claims, moral formation to orient goals, and strategic discomfort to toughen the system. Start small: sit for ten minutes, choose one negative thought, write a counter-statement, and do that every day. That single habit, practiced daily, is how a sound mind grows. Stand on business. Be merciless with the things that drag you down. Be merciful with yourself while you learn. Keep showing up.

Stand on business. The Spirit gives you power, love, and a sound mind. Not because you're special, but because God is generous. Ask for wisdom. Build the practices. Cut the toxicity. Teach the next generation. Your mind is worth the work. The people who depend on you are counting on it. So keep showing up.

CHAPTER THREE
A STRONG AND HEALTHY BODY

"What, know ye not that your body is the temple of the Holy Ghost which is in you . . . Therefore glorify God in your body and in your spirit, which are God's"

(1 Corinthians 6:19–20).

UNDERSTANDING A STRONG AND HEALTHY BODY

I was always athletic. Played sports growing up (track), moved well, had decent coordination. But I was short and skinny. No matter how much I ate or how active I stayed, I couldn't put on size. I didn't think much about it until my wife got pregnant with our oldest son.

That's when something shifted. I was about to be a dad, and I wanted to be the strong dad. Not just present, not just capable, but physically strong. The kind of dad who could carry his kid without getting winded, who could protect his family if needed, who looked like someone you didn't mess with. That mattered to me.

So I started lifting weights. I'd lifted weights before, but it was never consistently, and it was only because other friends or teammates were. I took it seriously this time, not just playing around. I was too embarrassed to walk into the gym, so I set up shop at home. I had a stability ball and ten-pound dumbbells and used them for everything: presses, rows, squats. Ten pounds. That's where I started. Let me tell you, I. Put. In. Work. I still have those ten-pound dumbbells. They hold sentimental value. Eventually, I made it to the gym because I needed more weight to lift.

Over the next few years, I put on forty pounds of lean muscle (waist size didn't change) using tried-and-true techniques. Nothing fancy. Progressive overload. Compound movements. Adequate protein. Consistency. The weight went up, the reps went up, and my body responded. I wasn't skinny anymore. I was jacked.

And I was in the mirror constantly. I loved how I looked. I'd catch my reflection in store windows, bathroom mirrors, anywhere I could see the progress. The shoulders got wider. The arms filled out. The chest built up. Legs were becoming trunks. Thighs were horse-like. It felt good. It felt like I'd finally achieved something I couldn't do naturally.

A couple of workout friends noticed. They suggested I do a bodybuilding show. At first, I laughed it off. But the idea stuck. I started researching, watching videos, studying posing routines. Eventually, I committed. I prepped for my first show, stepped on stage, and fell in love with it. It also urged me along, the fact that I won my first two shows.

That's when muscle building shifted from effort to art form. I became enamored with the idea that I could mold and shift my body through dedication and hard work. I loved how muscles layered on top of each other, how symmetry and proportion mattered as much as size, how deliberate training could sculpt specific areas. It wasn't just about being big. It was about being balanced, refined, intentional. My body became a canvas, and every workout was another brushstroke. I still feel this way.

But somewhere along the way, my perspective shifted again. I started seeing my body not just as art but also as something sacred. An important structure that houses the Spirit of God. I couldn't tell you when the shift actually happened. But it became apparent to me that this body isn't mine to do with as I please. It's a temple. God dwells in me. That changed everything, again. Caring for my body wasn't just about aesthetics anymore. It wasn't even just about craftsmanship. It was about stewardship. I was responsible for maintaining the physical platform where my mind, heart, and soul operate. Neglecting it wasn't humility.

It was a form of disobedience.

I also started noticing something troubling in the Christian community. A lot of believers were flat-out neglecting their bodies. I saw pastors burning out in their forties. Ministry leaders were sidelined by preventable health issues. Faithful servants' capacity to serve got cut short because they treated their bodies as expendable. They poured into everyone else while their own temple crumbled.

That's why this chapter exists. It's not to convince you to become a bodybuilder, not to shame you for being out of shape—not even to tell you that focusing on aesthetics is bad. This chapter exists to help you see what I finally saw: you can't ignore your body and expect the rest of your life to hold together. Caring for it isn't vanity. It's worship. And neglecting it isn't humility. It's poor stewardship that limits your capacity to do what God called you to do.

Here's the working definition: **a strong and healthy body is the physical platform where mind, heart, and soul operate.** Write that down. When the body is trained and healthy, your mind thinks clearer, your emotions stabilize, and your soul has the physical capacity to serve consistently. A neglected body produces brain fog, emotional volatility, and shortened service capacity. A strong body creates stamina, resilience, and extended years of faithful obedience.

This matters because if you want the rest of life to hold together over decades of relationships, ministry, leadership, and service, you start here. The body is not separate from your spiritual life. It is the physical structure through which spiritual life is lived out. Training the body is training for discipleship.

"As iron sharpens iron, so one person sharpens

another"(Proverbs 27:17).

Apply that principle internally: as iron sharpens iron, so a strong and healthy body sharpens your mind, heart, and soul. The process of building physical strength builds character, and the character you build physically transfers everywhere else.

HOW THIS CONNECTS TO SCAL

Your body determines how long you can show up. That's the bottom line. You can have a regulated heart, a sharp mind, and deep spiritual practices, but if your body breaks down, you're sidelined. The body is the physical structure that carries everything else, and when it fails, capacity disappears.

Physical training stabilizes your heart. Chronic stress from a weak, neglected body wrecks emotional regulation. Cortisol stays elevated. Sleep deteriorates. Anxiety compounds. But when you train consistently, the body's stress response recalibrates. Your nervous system learns to handle activation and recovery. The heart steadies because the body knows how to process stress instead of drowning in it.

Physical training sharpens your mind. Exercise increases BDNF, a protein that strengthens neural connections and supports brain plasticity. It improves blood flow to the brain, delivering more oxygen and clearing metabolic waste faster. The result is clearer thinking under pressure, faster learning when acquiring new skills, and better focus during long decision-making sessions.

Physical training extends your soul's capacity. Spiritual disciplines require endurance. Prayer demands sustained attention. Service demands physical presence over years, not months. A weak body gives out early. A strong body sustains the work. The discipline you build in the gym transfers to the discipline you need in the prayer closet. They're not separate. They're integrated.

Train the body, and everything else gains runway. Neglect the body, and everything else loses capacity.

PRACTICE PROMPT

❖ Write one sentence defining "strong and healthy body" in your own words.

❖ Then list one area of life, your work, your relationships, or your ministry, where physical strength would extend your capacity to serve.

Success Criteria

☐ You wrote your definition.
☐ You identified the specific area where physical strength would change outcomes.
☐ You read it aloud with conviction.
☐ Within twenty-four hours, you texted it to someone who knows you well.

Troubleshooting

If you can't bring yourself to text it, ask why. That resistance reveals how much you're performing versus how honest you're willing to be. If the person you texted responded with something generic, you picked the wrong person. Find someone who will actually call you on your patterns, not just affirm you.

TEMPLE STEWARDSHIP

Your body is the temple of the Holy Spirit. This is not metaphor. It is reality. The temple in Scripture was crafted with care, decorated to reflect God's glory, maintained as holy ground, and used as the central place where God and humanity met.

Your body carries the same dignity. God dwells in you through his Spirit. The care you give your body is worship. The neglect you allow is disobedience.

When Paul calls the body a temple, he's drawing on a rich theological foundation. The temple was crafted by skilled artisans. Your body is fearfully and wonderfully made, as Psalm 139:14 declares. The temple was set apart as holy. You are holy because God dwells in you. The temple required daily care through offerings, cleansing, and repair. Your body requires that same deliberate maintenance. The temple was used for worship and service. Your body is the instrument through which you serve.

Caring for the temple is about honoring the one who dwells within and preparing yourself to serve him longer. Solomon's temple had gold, fine wood, skilled craftsmanship. Artistry and craftsmanship honored God. But the moment people worshiped the building instead of the God who dwelt in it, judgment came. Build your temple with care, but keep the owner central. Let service be the fruit that proves your motive.

Here's the tension you must navigate: you must care for your body without making it an idol. The line is real. Bodybuilding can become narcissism. Training can become performance religion. Fitness can become your identity instead of a tool for service.

The guardrail is purpose. Ask yourself why you train. If the answer is "to look good" or "to prove something," you're in danger. If the answer is "to steward the temple and extend my capacity to serve," you're on track.

Craig's Two Paths

Craig is thirty-five years old with a desk job he's held for five years. He's sedentary, busy, and convinced he'll start training when things calm down. But when do things ever calm down?

Here's what happens if Craig keeps waiting.

Year one becomes year two, then three, then five. He's too busy for training, sleeping five hours a night, eating on the run. "I'll start when work slows down," he tells himself. But work never slows down.

By year six, the fatigue has become chronic. He's gained thirty pounds. His joints ache when he plays with his kids. At his annual physical, the doctor shows him a prediabetes diagnosis and suggests medication. Craig nods, promises to make changes, and does nothing.

By year ten, he can't play with his kids without getting winded. His back gives out when he tries to help a friend move. He's on three medications now. His wife notices he's irritable, exhausted, and always complaining about something hurting. Ministry commitments start slipping. He can't sustain the pace he once could. He tells himself it's just because he's getting older, but he's only forty-five.

By year fifteen, he's burned out. He takes a medical leave from work. Craig just can't serve in the ways he used to. His capacity has been cut short by preventable neglect. He had ten productive years, maybe fifteen if he pushed hard, and then breakdown. The temple wasn't maintained. The platform collapsed.

Imagine that Craig made a different choice.

He has the same job, the same busyness, and the same five-year starting point. But this time, Craig protects three training sessions per week. He's still busy, but he treats training like a meeting he can't cancel. He prioritizes seven to eight hours of sleep most nights. He eats clean enough—not perfect, but intentional. He's not chasing aesthetics. He's maintaining the temple.

By year six, he's still strong. His energy stays steady throughout the day. He handles long ministry commitments without crashing. His kids see discipline modeled in real time, not just talked about. At year ten, he's still sustaining the pace. He serves well. He disciples others. His physical capacity allows consistent service without breakdown. He's planning for another twenty productive years, not hoping to survive five more.

By year fifteen, he's still going. Craig is stronger than most men his age. He's still serving, still engaged, still present. The temple was maintained. The platform held.

Same calling. Different stewardship. The first approach treated the body as expendable and paid the price in shortened service. The second approach treated the body as the platform for long obedience and multiplied capacity over time.

Stewardship is not selfish. It's strategic. You can't serve from an empty tank or a broken temple. Every hour you invest in physical care extends your capacity to love, lead, and give over decades.

PRACTICE PROMPT

❖ Write one specific way your body's current condition limits your ability to serve. Be honest. You might say, "I can't help friends move because my back gives out" or "I'm too tired after work to engage with my kids" or "I avoid ministry opportunities because I don't have the stamina."

❖ Then commit to one training session this week as an act of stewardship, not vanity.

Success Criteria

☐ You identified a specific limitation.
☐ You scheduled one training session within the next seven days.
☐ You completed that session, and journaled afterward: "How does this prepare me to serve better?"

Troubleshooting

If you couldn't identify a limitation, either you're lying to yourself, or you're already in excellent shape. Ask your spouse or close friend what they see.

If you scheduled the session but didn't complete it, your commitment to stewardship is theoretical, not actual.

If you trained but couldn't articulate how it prepares you to serve, you're still treating fitness as separate from discipleship. Try again.

FOR HEART, MIND, AND SOUL

Training your body is not just about your body. A strong body benefits the heart, mind, and soul. Physical training upgrades your brain, stabilizes your emotions, and creates the stamina for sustained spiritual work. The connections are not metaphorical. They are biological.

Sharper Thinking Through Movement

A trained body changes the literal structure and function of your brain. Exercise increases BDNF, which strengthens synaptic connections and supports neuroplasticity. It improves blood flow to the brain, delivering more oxygen and glucose while clearing metabolic waste faster. It reduces chronic low-grade inflammation that slows processing speed and impairs executive function.

The result is that you think clearer on hard days, learn faster when acquiring new skills, and maintain focus under pressure.

Craig's Two-Hour Meeting

Craig has a critical strategic planning meeting on Tuesday afternoon. Two hours of complex information, competing priorities, and real-time decisions. Here's how two different physical states handle the same cognitive demand.

Sedentary Craig

Sedentary Craig hasn't trained in five years. The first thirty minutes of the meeting, he's mentally present, taking notes.

By the second thirty minutes, he's starting to fade. He's losing the thread. Drifting.

The third thirty minutes, he's struggling. Craig can't hold competing ideas simultaneously, and he gets irritable.

The final thirty minutes, he's checked out, nodding but not processing. He'll need a recap later.

Post-meeting, he's exhausted. Brain fog kills his afternoon. Poor recall nags at him.

Trained Craig

Trained Craig maintains three to four training sessions per week and has for the past two years. It's the same meeting with a different result. He's mentally present for the full two hours. Taking notes throughout is easy. Craig tracks multiple priorities simultaneously. He asks clarifying questions. Contributing meaningfully is effortless.

Post-meeting, he's tired but functional. Brain fog is minimal. He remembers key details and can act on them immediately.

Same person. Same meeting. Different physical preparation.

The trained brain has more metabolic capacity, better waste clearance, and stronger neural efficiency.

That's not motivational talk. That's physiology.

EMOTIONAL STEADINESS

Physical training regulates the nervous system, and the nervous system governs emotional response. When you train consistently, you teach your body to handle stress activation and recovery cycles. That skill transfers directly to emotional regulation.

Training also lowers baseline cortisol, the stress hormone that keeps you on edge. Chronic elevated cortisol wrecks sleep, amplifies anxiety, and makes every small trigger feel catastrophic. Consistent exercise brings cortisol back into normal range, which stabilizes mood and emotional reactivity.

Craig Receiving Critical Feedback

Craig gets critical feedback from his supervisor. Here's how two versions respond.

Sedentary Craig

Sedentary Craig's nervous system is dysregulated from years of inactivity and poor sleep. The feedback lands. His heart rate spikes immediately. His hands shake and his face flushes. He feels attacked, even though the feedback is fair. He responds defensively, voice raised, before he's thought it through.

He stews on it for three days. Craig can't sleep. He replays the conversation obsessively. The emotional charge doesn't fade. It compounds.

Trained Craig

Trained Craig's nervous system has been conditioned through repeated stress-recovery cycles in training. It's the same feedback and supervisor. His heart rate elevates but not to panic levels. He notices the physical response, names it internally as activation, and pauses before speaking.

He takes a breath, then asks a clarifying question. Craig thanks his supervisor for the input, says he'll think about it and follow up tomorrow.

Later that evening, he processes the feedback calmly with his wife.

By the next morning, the emotional charge has dissipated. He adjusts and moves forward.

It's the same feedback, but a different physical foundation. The trained nervous system knows how to return to baseline. The untrained nervous system stays stuck in activation.

Endurance That Transfers Everywhere

Physical endurance teaches spiritual endurance. The ability to push through discomfort in a workout builds the same capacity you need to sustain prayer, to serve when you're tired, to show up when you don't feel like it.

Every time you override the voice that says "quit early," you're building the override reflex. That reflex doesn't stay in the gym. It transfers to your prayer life, your relationships, your work, your ministry. The discipline to finish what you start physically becomes the discipline to finish what you start spiritually.

Craig's Prayer Commitment

Craig commits to pray for thirty minutes every morning. Here's how different levels of physical discipline affect that commitment.

Sedentary Craig has never built physical endurance. He's never trained himself to push through discomfort for a sustained period. When he sits down to pray, the first ten minutes are fine. By minute fifteen, his mind wanders. By minute twenty, he's restless, uncomfortable, looking for an excuse to stop. He tells himself he's done enough and quits at twenty-two minutes. The next day, he quits at eighteen. The pattern compounds. Within two weeks, he's down to five minutes and feeling guilty.

Trained Craig has built endurance in the gym. He knows what it feels like to hit the wall and keep going. He's conditioned his mind to override the quit signal. When he sits down to pray, the first ten minutes are fine. By minute fifteen, his mind wanders, just like sedentary Craig. By minute twenty, he's restless. But here's the difference: he recognizes the discomfort as part of the process. He's felt this in workouts. He knows it passes if he stays with it. He refocuses, keeps going, and finishes the full thirty minutes. The next day, it's slightly easier. The pattern compounds in the other direction. Within two weeks, thirty minutes feels normal.

It's the same commitment but a different capacity. Physical endurance builds the mental and spiritual capacity to sustain disciplines when they get hard.

PRACTICE PROMPT

❖ Pick one arena where you know a stronger body would help: sharper thinking during long meetings, steadier emotions under stress, or sustained endurance in spiritual practices.

❖ Write down one specific recent example where your current physical state limited you in that arena. Be detailed. What happened? How did your body respond? What did you have to stop or avoid because you didn't have the capacity?

❖ Then write one training commitment you'll make this week to start building that capacity.

Success Criteria

☐ You identified a specific limitation with concrete details.
☐ You wrote down one training commitment with a day and time scheduled.
☐ You completed that session within seven days and journaled afterward on whether you noticed any difference in the arena you targeted.

Troubleshooting

If you can't identify a limitation, you're either already in excellent shape or you're blind to how your physical state affects everything else. Ask your spouse or a close friend where they see your body limiting you.

If you identified the limitation but didn't schedule the session, you're treating this as theory instead of practice.

If you scheduled but didn't complete it, your stated priorities don't match your actual priorities.

If you completed the session but saw no difference, one session isn't enough. Commit to four weeks before evaluating.

THE TRAINING FRAMEWORK

Your body doesn't get stronger during training. It gets stronger during recovery after training. That distinction matters because most people overtrain or under-recover, and both wreck progress.

Training

Training is the stimulus. You stress the system. You break down muscle fibers, deplete energy stores, fatigue the nervous system. That breakdown is necessary, but it's not the goal. The goal is adaptation, and adaptation happens when you recover well.

Recovery

Recovery is where the magic happens. Sleep repairs tissue. Nutrition refills energy stores. Rest allows the nervous system to recalibrate. If you train hard but recover poorly, you don't adapt. You accumulate damage. Performance declines. Injury risk increases. The body breaks down instead of building up.

Adaptation

Adaptation is the result of adequate stimulus plus adequate recovery. Your body says, "That was hard. I need to be stronger next time." It builds more muscle, denser bones, better cardiovascular capacity, and improved neural efficiency. But only if you give it the resources and time to do so.

Repetition

Then you repeat the cycle. New stimulus. Better recovery. Stronger adaptation. Over weeks, months, and years, this compounds into a body that can handle more, last longer, and serve better.

Most people focus only on the training part. They chase harder workouts, more volume, greater intensity. But they neglect sleep, eat poorly, skip rest days, and wonder why their progress stalls. The framework isn't just to train harder. It's to train smart, recover intentionally, and let adaptation happen.

Training Volume and Intensity

Volume is how much work you do. Sets, reps, distance, duration. Intensity is how hard that work is. Heavy weight, fast pace, maximal effort. Both matter. Too little of either, and you don't create enough stimulus to force adaptation. Too much of either, and you exceed your recovery capacity.

The sweet spot depends on your current fitness level, your recovery capacity, and your goals. A beginner might need three training sessions per week at moderate intensity. An experienced lifter might handle five sessions with varied intensity. An endurance athlete might train six days with different volume and intensity targets each day.

The principle stays the same: match stimulus to recovery capacity. If you're constantly sore, fatigued, irritable, or experiencing declining performance, you've exceeded capacity. If you're not progressing after several weeks of consistent effort, you're not creating enough stimulus.

PRACTICE PROMPT

- ❖ Track your sessions.

- ❖ Notice patterns.

- ❖ Adjust accordingly.

Progressive Overload

Adaptation requires progression. If you do the same workout at the same intensity every week, your body has no reason to adapt. You've already adapted to that stimulus. Progress stops.

Progressive overload means gradually increasing the demand over time. Add weight to the bar. Add reps to the set. Add distance to the run. Decrease rest periods. Increase training frequency. The method varies, but the principle doesn't: do slightly more than last time.

The key word is *slightly*. Progression doesn't mean jumping from ten pushups to fifty pushups in one week. It means going from ten to twelve. Then twelve to fifteen. Then fifteen to eighteen. Small, consistent increases compound into significant strength over months.

Most people progress too aggressively and get injured or don't progress at all and plateau. Find the sustainable middle, which is enough to force adaptation, not so much that recovery fails.

PRACTICE PROMPT

❖ Review your last two weeks of physical activity. Did you train consistently? Did you progress in any measurable way, more weight, more reps, longer distance, better form? Did you recover well between sessions?

❖ Write down one specific progression you'll make this week. "I'll add five pounds to my squat" or "I'll run an extra quarter mile" or "I'll do one more set."

Success Criteria

☐ You reviewed your last two weeks honestly and identified whether you've been progressing or plateauing.
☐ You wrote down one specific progression target for this week.
☐ You executed that progression and noted whether it felt appropriately challenging or too aggressive.

Troubleshooting

If you haven't trained in the last two weeks, you're not ready to think about progression. You need to establish consistency first.

If you've trained but haven't progressed in months, you're coasting. Add stimulus.

If you tried to progress but got injured or excessively sore, you jumped too aggressively. Scale back, then progress more gradually.

BUILDING THE PLATFORM

Strength is the base physical quality. Everything else builds on it. Cardiovascular endurance, mobility, power, agility, all require a foundation of strength. Without it, you're limited in what you can do and how long you can sustain it.

Strength training stresses the musculoskeletal system, forcing muscles, tendons, ligaments, and bones to adapt. Over time, muscles grow denser and stronger. Tendons thicken. Ligaments stabilize joints better. Bone density increases. The nervous system learns to recruit muscle fibers more efficiently. The result is a body that can handle greater loads, resist injury, and perform tasks that would otherwise be impossible.

The benefits extend beyond the gym. Strength protects against age-related muscle loss (sarcopenia), which begins in your thirties and accelerates after age fifty. Strength improves metabolic health by increasing lean muscle mass, which burns more calories at rest and improves insulin sensitivity. Strength reduces chronic pain by stabilizing joints and correcting muscular imbalances. Strength extends independence in later years, allowing you to move, serve, and live without assistance.

Compound Movements vs. Isolation Work

Compound movements involve multiple joints and muscle groups working together. Squats, deadlifts, presses, rows, pull-ups are examples. These movements mimic real-world tasks and recruit the most muscle in the least time. They're efficient, functional, and produce the greatest hormonal response for muscle growth and strength gains.

Isolation movements target a single muscle group. Bicep curls, leg extensions, calf raises are some examples. These movements have their place for addressing weaknesses, correcting imbalances, or adding volume to specific muscles. But they shouldn't form the core of your training.

Prioritize compound movements. Build your program around squats, deadlifts, presses, and rows. Add isolation work as needed for weak points or aesthetic goals, but don't reverse the priority. Compound movements give you the most return on your training time.

Frequency and Recovery

Strength develops when you stress the muscle, recover adequately, and repeat. Frequency matters. Training a muscle group once a week provides minimal stimulus. Training it two to three times per week, with adequate recovery between sessions, produces better results.

Recovery between sessions depends on intensity and volume. Heavy, high-intensity sessions require more recovery time. Lighter, higher-volume sessions may allow shorter recovery windows.

Listen to your body. If you're consistently sore, fatigued, or experiencing declining performance, you need more recovery. If you're progressing steadily without excessive soreness, your frequency is appropriate.

Most people benefit from full-body training three times per week or an upper/lower split four times per week. Advanced lifters might handle more frequent training with careful programming. Beginners should start with three days and build from there.

Starting Points for Different Levels

If you're new to strength training, start simple. Learn the basic movements with light weight or bodyweight. Focus on form, not load. Squat, hinge, press, pull. Master these patterns before adding significant weight.

As I said earlier, I started off with ten-pound dumbbells. It was light, but I did ten sets of ten of every exercise. I don't suggest starting with so much volume. I just wanted to master those movements, so I had to "rep it out."

A beginner program might look like this:

- Three full-body sessions per week
- Five to six compound movements per session
- Three sets of eight to twelve reps per movement
- Progressing by adding reps, then weight, gradually

If you've been training consistently for a year or more, you can handle more volume and intensity. Split routines, varied rep ranges, and periodization become useful. But the principles stay the same: progressive overload, adequate recovery, consistency over time.

If you're returning after a long break, resist the urge to jump back in where you left off. Your strength will return faster than you expect, but your connective tissues need time to adapt. Start lighter than you think you should. Build back gradually. Avoid injury by respecting the adaptation timeline.

BUILDING THE ENGINE

Cardiovascular training strengthens the heart, improves oxygen delivery to tissues, and builds metabolic efficiency. It extends your capacity to sustain effort over time, whether that's running a 5K, playing with your kids without getting winded, or serving through a long ministry day without crashing.

Cardio comes in two primary forms: steady-state and high-intensity interval training. Both have value. Both should be part of a balanced program.

Steady-State Cardio

Sustained effort at a moderate intensity creates steady-state cardio. Running, cycling, swimming, or rowing at a pace you can maintain for twenty to sixty minutes are examples of steady-state cardio. Your heart rate stays elevated but steady. You can hold a conversation, but it's not easy.

Steady-state cardio builds aerobic capacity, the foundation of endurance. It improves mitochondrial density, which increases your cells' ability to produce energy efficiently. It enhances capillary networks, delivering more oxygen to working muscles. It strengthens the heart's ability to pump blood with each beat.

For most people, two to three steady-state sessions per week, twenty to forty minutes each, is sufficient. You don't need to run marathons to gain the benefits. Consistency at moderate effort beats sporadic heroic efforts.

High-Intensity Interval Training (HIIT)

This form of exercise alternates short bursts of maximal or near-maximal effort with rest or low-intensity recovery periods. Think sprints, bike intervals, rowing sprints, and sled pushes. Work hard for thirty seconds to two minutes, recover for one to three minutes, repeat.

This builds power, speed, and anaerobic capacity. It improves VO2 max, the maximum amount of oxygen your body can use during intense exercise. It burns significant calories in less time than steady-state cardio. It creates an afterburn effect, elevated calorie burn for hours post-workout.

One to two HIIT sessions per week is enough for most

because HIIT is demanding. It requires full recovery between sessions. More than one or two sessions per week, and you risk overtraining, especially if you're also strength training.

Balancing Cardio with Strength

Cardio supports strength training by improving recovery capacity and work tolerance. But excessive cardio interferes with strength gains by competing for recovery resources and creating conflicting adaptation signals.

The balance depends on your goals. If strength is the priority, keep cardio moderate. Two to three sessions per week at low to moderate intensity. If endurance is the priority, you can handle more cardio volume, but you'll need to reduce strength training volume to recover adequately.

Most people benefit from a balanced approach: three strength sessions, two to three cardio sessions, with at least one full rest day per week. Adjust based on your response and your specific goals.

RANGE OF MOTION

Mobility is the ability to move joints through their full range of motion with control. It's different from flexibility, which is passive range. Mobility is active. It requires strength at end ranges, not just the ability to stretch into a position.

Mobility declines with age and inactivity. Joints stiffen. Muscles tighten. Movement becomes restricted. That restriction leads to compensations, which lead to imbalances, which lead to pain and injury. Maintaining mobility prevents that cascade.

Daily Mobility Work

Mobility work doesn't require long sessions. Ten to fifteen minutes daily is more effective than hour-long sessions once a week. Focus on the joints and movements you use most: hips, shoulders, thoracic spine, and ankles.

Incorporate mobility into your warmup before training. Hip circles, shoulder dislocates, spinal rotations, ankle mobilizations. Move through ranges slowly and with control. The goal is to prepare the joints for loaded work and maintain full range over time.

If you have specific restrictions, tight hips, limited shoulder mobility, stiff ankles, address them with targeted work. Spend extra time on problem areas. Progress gradually. Forced stretching leads to injury. Patient, consistent work leads to improvement.

Yoga and Movement Practices

Yoga, tai chi, and similar movement practices build mobility, body awareness, and breath control. They complement strength and cardio training by improving movement quality and mental focus.

You don't need to become a yogi. One or two sessions per week can improve mobility and provide active recovery. Choose practices that emphasize controlled movement and breath, not just passive stretching.

FUELING THE TEMPLE

You know the old adage, "You can't out-train a poor diet." Training creates the stimulus for adaptation, but nutrition provides the raw materials. Without adequate fuel, recovery fails. Without recovery, adaptation doesn't happen. Progress stalls.

Nutrition doesn't need to be complicated. You don't need to count every macro or weigh every meal (not that it's bad to do so). But you do need to understand the basics and apply them consistently.

Hydration as the Foundation

Before we talk about food, we need to talk about water. Hydration is non-negotiable, and most people are walking around chronically dehydrated without realizing it.

The old guidelines said six to eight cups a day. That was inadequate. Current recommendations suggest eleven cups for women and fifteen cups for men, which works out to roughly a gallon of water daily. But even that might not be enough if you're training hard.

Some people use the "half your body weight in ounces" rule. If you weigh 150 pounds, you'd drink 75 ounces of water. That won't cut it, especially if you're athletic or doing any kind of serious training. Here's why: say you're that 150-pound person drinking 75 ounces daily. You train for an hour. Guidelines suggest adding twelve ounces of water per half hour of exercise. That's only twenty-four more ounces. You're still nowhere near what you're losing in sweat or what your body actually needs.

For active males, start with a gallon a day. For active females, start with ninety ounces daily. Then adjust based on how much you sweat, how hard you train, and how you feel. If your urine is dark yellow, you're dehydrated. Light yellow to clear means you're hydrated. It's that simple.

Here is a word of caution: there is such a thing as drinking too much water. Overhydration dilutes sodium levels in your blood, a condition called hyponatremia, which can be dangerous. If you're forcing down water to the point of nausea or your urine is completely clear all day, you've gone too far. Listen to your body. Thirst is a reliable signal. Drink consistently throughout the day, but don't turn hydration into an extreme sport.

Why does hydration matter this much? Your body uses water to transport nutrients and oxygen through your blood to working muscles. It uses water to clear metabolic waste from fatigued tissues. Every cellular process requires adequate hydration. When you're dehydrated, everything slows down. Nutrient delivery suffers. Waste removal lags. Recovery stalls.

If you're using any supplementation, protein shakes, creatine, pre-workout, anything, you need even more water. There was a study that claimed protein shakes lead to kidney stones. When you dig into the details, the issue wasn't the protein. It was dehydration. The people in the study weren't drinking enough water to process the protein load. Hydration matters even more when you're increasing protein intake or using supplements.

Water also keeps your joints lubricated, your skin healthy, and your digestion moving. It's one of the most basic things you can do for your body, especially if you're trying to lose weight. I can't tell you how many people I've coached who had weight-loss goals but drank maybe one cup of water a day. That doesn't make sense. Help your body out. Drink water. The changes come faster when you're adequately hydrated.

And listen, I know some of you don't like drinking water. You have to suck it up. Sure, you can drink coffee or tea, but you know how much coffee a gallon a day is? That's not going to work. A gallon of tea a day? Unless you're brushing your teeth after every cup, you're going to have stained teeth. More importantly, those aren't substitutes. Drink water. Get used to it. Discipline yourself if you need to, but get water into your system.

Protein as the Building Blocks

Protein is essential for muscle repair and growth. Every training session breaks down muscle tissue. Protein provides the amino acids needed to rebuild stronger. Without adequate protein, you're tearing down without rebuilding.

Aim for 0.8 to 1 gram of protein per pound of body weight daily. If you weigh 180 pounds, that's 144 to 180 grams of protein. Spread it across three to four meals. Your body can only process so much protein at once. Consistent intake throughout the day is more effective than one massive meal.

Good sources: lean meats, fish, eggs, dairy, legumes, protein powder if needed. Prioritize whole foods. Supplements fill gaps; they don't replace real food.

Carbohydrates as the Fuel Source

Carbohydrates fuel high-intensity work. Your muscles store glycogen, the carbohydrate form that your body uses for energy during training. Deplete glycogen without refilling it, and performance drops.

The amount you need depends on training volume and intensity. If you're training hard four to five days per week, you need more carbs than someone training twice per week at moderate intensity.

Focus on whole food sources: rice, potatoes, oats, fruits, vegetables. These provide energy plus vitamins, minerals, and fiber. Limit processed carbs and added sugars. They spike blood sugar, crash energy, and provide little nutritional value.

Fats as the Hormonal Regulator

Fats support hormone production, including testosterone, which is critical for muscle growth and recovery. They also provide long-term energy and support brain function.

Aim to obtain twenty to thirty percent of your total calories from fat. Prioritize healthy sources: olive oil, avocados, nuts, seeds, fatty fish. Limit trans fats and excessive saturated fats.

Nutrition Timing

When you eat matters, though less than most people think. Total daily intake matters more than precise timing. But strategic nutrition around training can support performance and recovery.

Before Training:

Two to three hours before your workout, eat a full meal: at least twenty-five grams of protein, complex carbs like rice or oats, and some healthy fats. This gives your body time to digest and convert food to usable energy.

If you're training early and can't eat a full meal hours beforehand, eat something lighter thirty to sixty minutes before: fast-digesting carbs like fruit, maybe some yogurt, a small smoothie. Keep it light so you don't feel sluggish or nauseous during training. Stay away from heavy fats close to your workout. They slow digestion and can cause discomfort.

Now here's the thing: for a normal strength workout, one hour or less, you don't necessarily need special fueling if you have a balanced diet. Your body has enough stored energy to handle that work. But if you're doing resistance training longer than ninety minutes, powerlifters do this, bodybuilders who train twice a day do this, you'll need proper fueling beforehand. The intensity and duration demand it.

You also want to consider fueling for HIIT workouts and endurance cardio. These deplete glycogen quickly. You're burning through muscle glycogen, then your liver starts converting its stores, and eventually you risk breaking down muscle tissue for fuel. You don't want that. Fuel those sessions with simple, fast-digesting carbs beforehand.

During Training

For most people doing normal one-hour sessions, water is all you need. Stay hydrated. That's it.

If you're doing extended resistance training, HIIT, or long endurance sessions, consider an electrolyte solution, especially if you sweat heavily. BCAAs (branch-chained amino acids) during workouts can aid endurance and reduce soreness, but they're not mandatory. Most people will be fine with just water.

After Training:

Post-workout nutrition jumpstarts recovery. After resistance training, protein is the priority. I drink protein shakes, and I start sipping mine toward the end of my workout, usually with two sets left in my last exercise. That way the recovery process begins immediately.

After a HIIT session, the focus shifts. You need a combination of simple carbs transitioning into complex carbs, plus protein. Start with fast-digesting carbs to replenish glycogen quickly, then move to complex carbs for sustained energy.

Two to three hours after training, eat a full meal: twenty-five grams of protein, complex carbs, healthy fats. This supports full recovery and prepares your body for the next session.

The Bottom Line

Don't overthink nutrition. Eat balanced meals throughout the day. Get protein at each meal. Fuel your training with carbs. Include healthy fats. Stay hydrated. Consistency beats perfection.

THE FOUNDATION OF RECOVERY

Sleep is where adaptation happens. Hormones reset. Tissues repair. The brain consolidates learning. Neglect sleep, and everything else suffers significantly.

Most adults need seven to nine hours per night. Some need more, especially if training intensely. Few truly function well on less, though many convince themselves they do.

Why Sleep Matters for Training

Better recovery from your workouts is connected to quality sleep. Sleep is when your body repairs broken-down muscle tissue and builds it back stronger. Skip sleep, and you're not recovering. You're accumulating damage.

You get an immune system boost. Chronic sleep deprivation wrecks immunity. You get sick more often, stay sick longer, and can't train consistently.

Sleep regulates leptin and ghrelin, the hormones that control hunger and metabolism. Poor sleep throws these off, making fat loss harder and muscle gain slower. Sleep also affects testosterone, cortisol, and growth hormone, all critical for recovery and adaptation.

Emotional regulation is easier. Sleep deprivation makes you irritable, anxious, and emotionally volatile. You know this if you've ever tried to function on four hours of sleep. Everything feels harder. Your patience disappears. Your heart becomes unstable.

It prevents injuries. Fatigued bodies move poorly. Reaction times slow. Coordination suffers. You're more likely to get hurt training on inadequate sleep than you are training well-rested.

Sleep provides stress relief. During sleep, your nervous system downshifts from sympathetic activation (fight or flight) to parasympathetic (rest and digest). Without adequate sleep, you stay stuck in stress mode.

Sleep Quality Markers

Quality matters as much as quantity. Deep sleep is where physical recovery happens. The rapid-eye movement (REM) phase of sleep is where mental and emotional processing occurs. Both are necessary.

These are signs of poor sleep quality: waking frequently, feeling unrefreshed in the morning, relying on caffeine to function, irritability, brain fog, declining performance in training.

If you're sleeping eight hours but still feel exhausted, your sleep quality is compromised. Address it.

How to Optimize Sleep

Build a rhythm.

Your body works in rhythms. Set your body on a timer. Go to sleep at the same time every night. Wake up at the same time every morning, even on weekends. Your circadian rhythm thrives on consistency. When you maintain that timing, your body knows when to produce melatonin, when to lower cortisol, and when to prepare for rest.

Manage caffeine and alcohol.

Stay away from caffeine and alcohol close to bedtime. You don't want eight cups of coffee before bed. You don't want twenty shots of something before bed. Both jack up your sleep. Caffeine has a half-life of five to six hours. Coffee at 3 PM is still in your system at 9 PM, interfering with sleep onset. Alcohol might help you fall asleep faster, but it wrecks deep sleep and REM cycles. Limit caffeine after early afternoon. Avoid alcohol close to bedtime.

Create the right environment.

Sleep in a dark, cold room. Studies show you're more likely to get better sleep in a chilled, dark environment. I personally sleep better in warmth. I love the heat, but the research says otherwise. So if you're struggling with sleep quality, try lowering the temperature.

There are also studies on room color. Purple is supposedly one of the worst colors for sleep. Gray or certain shades of blue are better. I don't know how much that matters, but it's worth considering.

Shut off screens.

If you work right up until bedtime, stop doing that. Use no tablets, no TVs, no phones, no e-readers for at least two hours before shuteye. Blue light from screens suppresses melatonin production, the hormone that makes you sleepy. Shut off screens well before bed. Start reducing the amount of light you see as you get closer to sleep. This helps your body build the routine for rest. Look for screen covers and apps that reduce blue light, such as F.lux

Get enough magnesium.

Magnesium supports better sleep. Dark leafy greens, nuts, and seeds are good sources. Make sure you're getting enough.

Exercise smart.

Exercise is important, but timing matters. The closer you get to bedtime, the less intense the exercise should be. You're not going to do a spin class ten minutes before bed. That's counterproductive.

Intense exercise elevates cortisol and activates your nervous system. You need time to downshift. If you train late, keep it moderate or focus on mobility work.

Establish a wind-down routine.

Create a buffer between the day's stress and sleep. Read an actual book, not an e-reader. Pray. Journal. Stretch. Do light mobility work. A lot of people have a stretching routine right before bed. It's calming, and it leads to better sleep. I used to do it for years.

Your nervous system needs time to downshift. Don't expect to go from full activation to deep sleep in five minutes. Build the transition.

If you wake up in the middle of the night, one of the worst things you can do is lie there staring at the ceiling. Don't do that. If you wake up and can't fall back asleep within fifteen minutes, get up. Move around a little. Restart your night routine in condensed form. Read a book, sitting in a chair next to the bed. Do some light stretching. Then get back into bed.

You want your body to associate the bed with sleeping, not with lying awake frustrated. Train your body that when you're in bed, you should be sleeping.

Sleep position matters.

Sleep on your side, preferably your right side. Studies show this promotes better brain and heart health. When you sleep on your side, your brain's waste-clearance system works more efficiently. It gets rid of metabolic waste faster. Sleeping on your right side specifically jumpstarts the recovery process for your brain and heart.

Don't sleep on your back or your belly. Those positions don't promote good sleep quality and can cause issues over time. The exception is if you're late-term pregnant, sleep on your left side because your uterus is displacing your organs. But for everyone else, right side is best.

Sleep Deprivation and Training

Training on inadequate sleep is counterproductive. You won't perform well. You'll increase injury risk. Recovery will suffer. One or two nights of poor sleep won't destroy you, but chronic sleep deprivation will wreck progress. If you're sleep-deprived, adjust training intensity or skip the session entirely. Rest is productive. Exhaustion is not.

PRACTICE PROMPT—PART 1:

❖ Audit your current training, nutrition, and sleep for seven consecutive days.

- **Track your training:** How many days did you train? What modalities (strength, cardio, mobility)? Did you progress in any measurable way—weight, reps, distance, better form?

- **Track your nutrition:** Did you hit your protein target daily (0.8–1g per pound of bodyweight)? Were carbs and fats balanced around your training? Did you stay adequately hydrated?

- **Track your sleep:** How many hours did you get per night? Did you wake feeling refreshed or exhausted? Was your sleep schedule consistent?

❖ At the end of the week, identify your weakest area. Write down one specific change you'll make in that area for the following week.

Success Criteria

☐ You tracked all three areas for seven full days.
☐ You identified which area needs the most attention based on actual data (not assumption).
☐ You made one specific improvement in that area and executed that change for at least five out of the next seven days.

Troubleshooting

If tracking for a full week feels impossible, you're likely overcomplicating it. Use simple metrics: training days (yes/no), approximate protein intake, hours slept. Perfect tracking isn't the goal; awareness is.

If you tracked everything but can't identify a weakness, compare your current habits against the guidelines in each section. Gaps will become obvious.

If you identified the weakness but didn't follow through with changes, your commitment is theoretical rather than actual. Start smaller—one training session, twenty more grams of protein daily, or thirty more minutes of sleep. Build from there.

TOOLS BEYOND THE BASICS

Sleep, nutrition, and rest days form the foundation of recovery. But additional modalities can accelerate adaptation, reduce soreness, and extend your training capacity. These aren't necessary for everyone, but they are worth understanding if you're training hard and want every advantage.

Sauna Therapy

Heat exposure through sauna use triggers multiple beneficial adaptations. Regular sauna sessions improve cardiovascular function, increase heat shock proteins that protect cells from stress, enhance blood flow, and promote detoxification through sweat.

Research shows that consistent sauna use, four to seven sessions per week at 174–212°F for fifteen to twenty minutes, reduces the risk of cardiovascular disease and all-cause mortality. The heat stress mimics moderate cardiovascular exercise, increasing heart rate and blood flow without the mechanical stress on joints and muscles.

Heat shock proteins, produced during heat exposure, protect cells from damage and support muscle repair. They help prevent protein degradation and improve cellular resilience. Over time, regular heat exposure makes you more tolerant to physical stress, both in training and in daily life.

Post-workout sauna sessions aid recovery by increasing blood flow to fatigued muscles, accelerating waste removal and nutrient delivery. The relaxation effect also helps regulate the nervous system, shifting from sympathetic (stress) to parasympathetic (rest and digest) activation.

Start conservatively if you're new to sauna use. Begin with ten to twelve minutes at moderate heat. Build tolerance gradually. Stay hydrated. Exit if you feel dizzy or nauseated. Consistency matters more than duration. Three to four sessions per week at fifteen minutes beats one heroic thirty-minute session that leaves you depleted.

Cold Exposure

Cold exposure, through ice baths, cold plunges, or cold showers, triggers different adaptations than heat. Cold reduces inflammation and soreness post-training, activates brown fat, which improves metabolic health, and builds mental resilience by forcing you to override discomfort.

Mechanism

The mechanism is simple. Cold constricts blood vessels, reducing blood flow to inflamed areas. When you warm up afterward, blood flow returns rapidly, flushing metabolic waste and delivering fresh nutrients. This cycle accelerates recovery.

Cold also activates brown adipose tissue, a type of fat that burns calories to generate heat. Regular cold exposure increases brown fat activity, improving metabolic function and insulin sensitivity over time.

The mental benefit is significant. Stepping into cold water requires overriding your nervous system's immediate protest. That override builds the same discipline you need in training, in relationships, in spiritual practices. Discomfort becomes familiar. You learn to stay calm in activation. That skill transfers everywhere.

Timing

Timing matters with cold exposure. Immediately post-strength training, cold can blunt the inflammatory response needed for muscle growth. If your goal is hypertrophy, wait three to four hours after lifting before cold exposure. If your goal is recovery from high-volume or endurance work, immediate cold helps.

Start with cold showers. Try thirty seconds at the end of your normal shower. Build to one to two minutes. Then progress to ice baths or cold plunges, two to four minutes at 50–60°F. Don't force heroic efforts. Build tolerance gradually.

Red Light Therapy (Photobiomodulation)

Red light therapy uses specific wavelengths of light, 600–900 nanometers, to penetrate skin and stimulate cellular energy production. Mitochondria absorb the light and increase adenosine triphosphate (ATP) production, the energy currency of cells.

More ATP means faster recovery, reduced inflammation, and improved tissue repair.

Research supports red light therapy for reducing muscle soreness, accelerating wound healing, and improving skin health. Athletes use it to speed recovery between training sessions. The low-risk therapy is noninvasive and increasingly accessible.

Treatment duration varies by device intensity, but most protocols recommend ten to twenty minutes per session, three to five times per week, positioned six to twelve inches from the targeted area.

Red light therapy won't replace sleep or nutrition, but it can supplement recovery if you're training at high volume or dealing with chronic soreness or injury.

Hyperbaric Oxygen Therapy (HBOT)

Hyperbaric oxygen therapy involves breathing pure oxygen in a pressurized chamber. The increased pressure allows oxygen to dissolve into blood plasma at higher concentrations than normal breathing. That oxygen reaches tissues with compromised blood flow, accelerating healing and reducing inflammation.

This therapy is used medically for wound healing, carbon monoxide poisoning, and decompression sickness. Athletes use it to speed recovery from injury and reduce systemic inflammation from hard training.

Sessions typically last sixty to ninety minutes at one and a half to three times normal atmospheric pressure. Frequency depends on the person's goals: injury recovery might require daily sessions for weeks, while general recovery maintenance might use one to two sessions per week.

Because HBOT is expensive and not available in every town, it is less accessible than other recovery modalities. It's not necessary for most people. But if you're recovering from significant injury or training at elite levels, it's worth considering.

Massage and Soft-Tissue Work

Massage reduces muscle tension, improves circulation, and provides psychological relaxation. Deep tissue work, myofascial release, and trigger-point therapy address specific adhesions and restrictions that limit movement and cause pain.

You don't need weekly massages to benefit. Monthly sessions for maintenance, with more frequent visits during high-volume training blocks or when dealing with specific issues, provide value without excessive cost.

Self-myofascial release using foam rollers, lacrosse balls, or massage guns offers a more accessible alternative. Spend ten to fifteen minutes post-training targeting tight or sore areas. Roll slowly, pause on tender spots, breathe through the discomfort. This isn't a substitute for professional work, but it helps maintain tissue quality between sessions.

Compression Therapy

Compression garments and pneumatic compression devices improve circulation and reduce swelling post-training. They work by applying external pressure that helps push blood and lymph back toward the heart, clearing metabolic waste from fatigued muscles.

Research is mixed on performance benefits, but subjective reports of reduced soreness and faster recovery are common. Compression boots, the pneumatic devices that cycle pressure up the legs, are popular among endurance athletes and anyone dealing with significant leg fatigue.

If you have access to compression therapy, use it. If not, elevating your legs for ten to fifteen minutes post-training achieves a similar, though less-pronounced, effect.

Integration and Prioritization

You don't need all these modalities. Start with the basics: sleep, nutrition, rest days. If those are dialed in and you want additional recovery support, add one or two enhanced modalities based on the access and goals you have.

Sauna and cold exposure are the most accessible and provide

broad benefits. Massage and soft-tissue work address specific issues. Red light and HBOT are more specialized and expensive but useful for targeted recovery needs.

Don't let recovery tools become a distraction from consistent training. Recovery supports training. Training drives adaptation. Keep the priorities straight.

PRACTICE PROMPT — PART 2:

If you completed Part One and addressed your weakest recovery area, you're ready to consider enhanced recovery modalities. If you skipped Part One, go back and do it first. Enhanced recovery tools don't fix broken fundamentals.

❖ Assuming your basics are solid — consistent training, adequate protein and hydration, seven-plus hours of quality sleep — choose one enhanced modality to experiment with for two weeks:
  • Post-workout sauna sessions (three to four times per week, fifteen to twenty minutes)
  • Cold exposure after training (two to three times per week, starting with thirty-second cold showers)
  • Daily mobility work (ten to fifteen minutes)
  • Weekly massage or foam rolling sessions

❖ Track your recovery markers: soreness levels, sleep quality, training performance, mood for two weeks.

❖ At the end of two weeks, evaluate whether the modality made a measurable difference.

Success Criteria

□ You confirmed your basics are in place from Part One.
□ You chose one enhanced recovery practice.
□ You implemented it consistently (at least ten out of fourteen opportunities).
□ You tracked your recovery markers.
□ You can articulate whether it provided value worth continuing.

Troubleshooting

If you're tempted to skip Part One and jump straight to enhanced modalities, you're avoiding the harder work of fixing fundamentals. Time in a sauna won't fix chronic sleep deprivation. Cold plunges won't compensate for inadequate protein. Do the basics first.

If you try an enhanced modality but see no benefit, either your basics still need work, or that particular modality doesn't fit your needs. Try a different one, or accept that you might not need extras right now.

If consistency was the issue, the modality you chose might not be accessible enough. Cold showers are easier to sustain than gym sauna sessions. Start with what you can actually maintain.

STRATEGIC METABOLIC STRESS

Fasting is the voluntary abstention from food for a defined period. It's been practiced for thousands of years for spiritual, health, and practical reasons. Modern research confirms what ancient wisdom knew: fasting triggers beneficial metabolic adaptations when done correctly.

Fasting is not starvation. Starvation is involuntary, prolonged, and harmful. Fasting is controlled, temporary, and when done properly, beneficial.

Physiological Effects of Fasting

When you stop eating, your body shifts fuel sources. Insulin drops. Glucagon rises. The body starts breaking down glycogen stores for energy. After twelve to eighteen hours, glycogen depletes and the body shifts to fat metabolism, producing ketones for fuel.

This metabolic switch triggers a process called autophagy (pronounced aw-TAH-fuh-jee), meaning "self-eating." It is a cellular cleaning process where damaged proteins and organelles are broken down and recycled. Autophagy declines with age and constant feeding. Fasting reactivates it, improving cellular health and potentially extending lifespan.

Fasting also improves insulin sensitivity, reduces inflammation, and promotes growth hormone release, which supports muscle preservation during caloric restriction.

These benefits accumulate with consistent practice. Occasional fasting won't transform your health; regular, strategic fasting can.

Types of Fasting

Intermittent fasting restricts eating to a specific window each day. The most common protocol is 16:8, 16 hours fasting, 8 hours eating. You might eat between noon and 8 PM, fasting from 8 PM to noon the next day.

This pattern is sustainable for most people. You're sleeping through much of the fast. You skip breakfast, which some find easy, others find difficult. The eating window is long enough to get adequate calories and nutrients.

Other protocols include 18:6, 20:4, or even one meal a day (OMAD). More aggressive windows require more planning to ensure adequate nutrition. They're not inherently better. Sustainability matters more than extremity.

Extended fasting involves twenty-four hours or longer without food. A twenty-four-hour fast might run from dinner one day to dinner the next. Longer fasts of forty-eight to seventy-two hours amplify metabolic benefits but require more preparation and aren't necessary for most people.

Fasting and Training

Fasting while training requires careful timing. Strength training in a fasted state is possible but not ideal for performance or muscle growth. Your body needs fuel for maximal effort and protein for recovery.

If you're doing intermittent fasting, schedule training to take place during or near the end of your eating window. Eat protein and carbs post-workout to support recovery.

Low-intensity cardio in a fasted state is well-tolerated and may enhance fat oxidation (fat burning). High-intensity work suffers without fuel. Match training intensity to feeding state.

Extended fasts and hard training don't mix. If you're doing a multi-day fast, reduce training volume and intensity, or rest entirely. Recovery requires nutrients. You can't build without raw materials.

Spiritual Integration

Fasting has always been a spiritual practice. Jesus fasted. The early church fasted. Scripture commands fasting not as a meaningless ritual but as a tool for focused prayer and dependence on God.

Matthew 6:16–18 warns against performative fasting. Don't fast to be seen. Fast to seek God. The physical discipline of fasting creates space for spiritual focus. Hunger becomes a reminder to pray. Weakness becomes a reminder of dependence.

Isaiah 58 redefines fasting as more than abstaining from food. God's chosen fast includes justice, mercy, and care for the oppressed. Fasting without compassion is just dieting.

Fasting should be rooted in purpose. If you're fasting for metabolic benefits alone, fine, but you're missing the deeper practice. Fast to seek God. Let the physical hunger point you toward spiritual hunger. Let the discipline train dependence. Psalm 63:1 captures it:

"My soul thirsts for you; my flesh faints for you" (Psalm 63:1).

Fasting embodies that thirst physically. You feel it. You can't ignore it. That's the point. More on this in the next chapter.

Practical Fasting Guidelines

Start small. If you've never fasted, begin with a twelve-hour overnight fast. Then extend to fourteen, then sixteen. Build your tolerance gradually.

Stay hydrated. Water, black coffee, and unsweetened tea are acceptable during fasting windows. They don't break the fast, and they help manage hunger.

Break fasts gently. Don't go from a twenty-four-hour fast to a massive meal. Start with something light, protein and vegetables, then eat normally an hour or two later.

Listen to your body. If you feel weak, dizzy, or excessively irritable, eat. Fasting should be challenging, not dangerous. Some people tolerate fasting better than others. Find what works for you.

Avoid fasting if you're pregnant, nursing, underweight, or have a history of disordered eating. Fasting is a tool, not a requirement. It's not for everyone.

When Not to Fast

Fasting is not appropriate during high-volume training phases. You need fuel to perform and recover. Fasting while trying to build muscle is counterproductive. You can maintain muscle during fasting, but you won't build optimally.

Fasting is not a weight-loss magic bullet. It works for fat loss because it restricts eating time, which often reduces total calorie intake. If you binge during your eating window, you won't lose weight. Fasting helps, but it's not a substitute for reasonable nutrition.

Fasting is not penance. Don't fast to punish yourself for overeating. That's disordered thinking and disordered eating. Fast with purpose, for health or spiritual focus, not guilt.

PRACTICE PROMPT

Critical Instruction

Consult your doctor before attempting any fasting protocol. This is especially important if you have existing health conditions, take medications, are pregnant or nursing, have a history of disordered eating, or are currently underweight.

Fasting is not appropriate for everyone, and that's okay. This practice is optional, not mandatory.

- ❖ If you've never fasted and your doctor has cleared you to try it, attempt a twelve to sixteen-hour overnight fast. Stop eating after dinner. Don't eat again until late morning or lunch the next day. Drink water, coffee, or tea during the fasting window. If you have fasted before, do what you know works for you. No matter which group you are in, it's okay to start small.

- ❖ Journal your experience. What did you notice physically? Mentally? Spiritually? Did hunger feel overwhelming or manageable? Did you pray more? Think more clearly? Feel weak or lightheaded?

❖ After completing one fast, decide: Is this a practice worth continuing? If yes, commit to one or two fasting days per week for a month. If no, that's fine. Fasting isn't mandatory for stewardship.

Success Criteria

☐ You consulted a healthcare provider if you have any medical concerns.
☐ You completed one twelve- to sixteen-hour fast.
☐ You journaled your physical, mental, and spiritual observations with specific details (not "it was fine").
☐ You made a clear decision about whether to continue the practice based on your actual experience and medical guidance.

Troubleshooting

If your doctor advised against fasting due to medical conditions or medications, respect that guidance. Your health comes first, and there are other spiritual disciplines you can practice.

If you're cleared medically but couldn't make it twelve hours, assess why. True medical issues (dizziness, severe headaches, dangerous blood sugar drops) mean you should stop and consult your doctor. General discomfort or mild hunger is normal and manageable—that's part of the discipline.

If you fasted but didn't journal, you missed the opportunity for self-awareness. The point isn't just to skip meals; it's to observe what fasting reveals about your relationship with food, comfort, and God.

If you're uncertain whether fasting is right for you, start by asking your doctor rather than attempting it and hoping for the best. This isn't a practice to experiment with recklessly.

MISTAKES THAT WRECK PROGRESS

Most people fail not from lack of effort but from repeating the same mistakes that guarantee stagnation or injury. Knowing these patterns helps you avoid them.

Mistake One: Chasing Intensity Without Building Capacity

Beginners often try to train like advanced lifters. They see someone doing high-volume, high-intensity work and assume that's what they need to do. It's not. Advanced lifters earned that capacity over years. Their connective tissues adapted. Their nervous systems can handle the load. Yours can't, not yet.

Jumping into advanced programming leads to overtraining, injury, or burnout within weeks. You need progressive adaptation, starting light, building volume and intensity gradually over months and years.

Start with three training days per week at moderate intensity. Master basic movements with proper form. Add weight slowly. Build the foundation before trying to build the skyscraper.

Mistake Two: Ignoring Recovery Signals

Your body sends clear signals when recovery is inadequate. Persistent soreness that doesn't improve is one. Another is declining performance, such as lifts getting weaker, runs getting slower, and resting heart rate increasing. Irritability and mood swings are also common. Disrupted sleep and frequent minor illnesses are more signals.

These aren't signs to push harder. They're warnings to back off. Ignoring them leads to injury, illness, or complete breakdown.

Recovery is not weakness. It's strategy. Listen to the signals. Adjust volume, reduce intensity, add rest days, improve sleep, increase calories. Don't wait until you're forced to stop. Manage recovery proactively.

Mistake Three: Program Hopping

Every few weeks, you see a new program online. It promises better results, faster gains, the secret you've been missing. So you switch. Two weeks later, another program looks better. You switch again. Six months pass. You've tried eight programs. None of them worked.

The problem isn't the programs. The problem is the switching. Progress requires consistency over time. Every solid program works if you stay with it long enough. None of them works if you quit after two weeks.

Pick a reasonable program, one that matches your experience level and goals. Commit to it for at least twelve weeks. Track your progress. Adjust based on results, not boredom or shiny object syndrome.

Consistency beats novelty. Stay the course.

Mistake Four: Neglecting Mobility and Movement Quality

Strength without mobility creates dysfunction. You can squat heavy weight with compromised form, limited range, and compensatory patterns. That works until it doesn't. Then injury sidelines you.

Mobility work feels boring. It doesn't produce the same endorphin rush as heavy lifting or hard cardio. But it prevents the injuries that stop progress entirely.

Spend ten to fifteen minutes daily on mobility. Warm up properly before training. Address restrictions before they become problems. Movement quality matters as much as movement quantity.

Mistake Five: Training Through Pain

Discomfort is part of training. The burn of lactic acid, the fatigue of hard effort, soreness the next day are all normal. Pain is different. Sharp pain, joint pain, and pain that persists or worsens are all a signal to stop.

Training through pain doesn't build toughness. It builds injury. You're teaching your body to operate in dysfunction, which creates compensations that lead to bigger problems.

If something hurts, stop. Assess. Modify the movement. Reduce the load. Seek professional guidance if needed. Don't let pride turn a minor issue into a chronic problem.

Mistake Six: All-or-Nothing Thinking

You miss a workout. Life happens. Maybe it's an unexpected demand, a sick kid, or a legitimate emergency. Instead of adjusting and moving forward, you decide the whole week is ruined. You skip the next session, too. Then the next. One missed workout becomes a month off.

Or you eat poorly one meal. Instead of getting back on track at the next meal, you decide the day is blown. You binge the rest of the day, then the weekend. One bad meal becomes a week-long derailment.

This thinking wrecks consistency. Progress comes from what you do most of the time; you don't have to do something perfectly all the time to see progress. One missed workout is not failure. One poor meal is not disaster. Get back on track at the next opportunity. Keep moving forward.

Perfection is the enemy of progress. Consistency with occasional imperfection beats sporadic perfection every time.

Mistake Seven: Comparing

Don't compare your Chapter One to someone else's Chapter Twenty. You see someone lifting twice what you lift, running twice as far, looking twice as fit. You compare yourself and feel inadequate. You either quit because you'll never measure up, or you try to match their intensity and get injured.

Everyone started somewhere. That person you're comparing yourself to probably has years of training you can't see. They've built capacity you haven't built yet. Comparing their current state to your current state is pointless.

Compare yourself to yourself. Are you stronger than you were last month? Faster than you were last year? More consistent than before? That's the only comparison that matters.

Run your race. Build your capacity. Trust the process.

WARNING SIGNS

Training should make you better over time. If it's making you worse, something is wrong. Somtimes, you need to stop or seek help.

Physical Warning Signs

Be alert for persistent joint pain that doesn't improve with rest. Sharp, stabbing pain during movement, swelling that doesn't resolve, and numbness or tingling in extremities all require professional evaluation. Don't self-diagnose. Don't push through. See a doctor, physical therapist, or sports medicine specialist.

The following indicate overtraining or inadequate recovery:

- Chronic fatigue that doesn't improve with sleep
- Declining performance across multiple sessions
- Elevated resting heart rate for several consecutive days
- Frequent illness

Reduce training volume, improve sleep, increase calories, add rest days.

Sudden, significant weight loss or gain without dietary changes, changes in menstrual cycle for women, or loss of libido suggest hormonal disruption, possibly from overtraining or undereating. Address nutrition and recovery immediately.

Mental and Emotional Warning Signs

Loss of motivation that persists for weeks. Dreading workouts you used to enjoy. Irritability and mood swings. Anxiety around training. These often accompany overtraining but can also signal burnout or misaligned priorities.

Training should energize you over time, not drain you. If you're consistently exhausted, frustrated, or anxious about training, something needs to change. Reduce intensity, vary your routine, take a week off, or reassess your goals.

If training has become an obsession where missing a session creates intense guilt or anxiety, you've crossed into disordered territory. Training is a tool for stewardship, not an idol. If you can't rest without guilt, you need to examine your motives and potentially seek help.

When to Seek Professional Guidance

If you're new to training and don't know where to start, hire a coach or trainer. A few sessions to learn proper form and basic programming will save you months of frustration and potential injury.

If you're dealing with chronic pain or recurring injuries, see a physical therapist. Self-treating rarely works. Professional assessment identifies root causes and provides targeted solutions. If you've been training consistently for months without progress, your programming or nutrition likely needs adjustment.

A coach can identify blind spots and provide accountability.

If training is creating anxiety, obsession, or relationship conflict, talk to a counselor. Physical training should serve your whole life, not consume it.

FINAL WARNINGS: GUARDRAILS

Before we close, there are critical warnings that protect you from derailing or distorting the work.

Warning One: Stewardship is not elective.
If you want to serve God effectively, physical stewardship is not optional. Trials will come. Adversity will test you. If your body is weak, you'll break.

"But I keep under my body, and bring it into subjection:

lest that by any means, when I have preached to others,

I myself should be a castaway" (1 Corinthians 9:27).

Paul disciplined his body. He trained himself. Because he knew that without discipline, he could disqualify himself. The same applies to you.

You can't coast on spiritual disciplines alone while neglecting the physical platform that carries them. The body matters. Steward it.

Warning Two: Comfort is a slow poison.
The more comfortable you are, the weaker you become. Comfort atrophies everything: body, mind, heart, soul.

If your life is easy right now, thank God. Then introduce strategic discomfort before life introduces involuntary adversity. Train now so you're ready when trials come.

Your body doesn't care about your excuses. It responds to stimulus. Give it none, and it weakens. Give it progressive challenge, and it strengthens. The choice is yours, but the consequences are inevitable.

Warning Three: You will fail sometimes.
Some days, you'll quit the workout early. Some days, you'll skip entirely. Some days, you'll eat poorly. Some days, you'll neglect

recovery. That's not the end.

Get back up. Try again. Endurance is built through repeated effort, not perfection. Confess, receive grace, and return to the work.

Romans 12:1 says to present your bodies as a living sacrifice. Sacrifices aren't perfect. They're offered. Keep offering. Keep showing up. Faithfulness matters more than flawlessness.

Warning Four: Steward the temple without worshiping it. The line between stewardship and idolatry is real. Build your temple with care, but keep God central. Let service be the fruit that proves your motive.

If your training makes you proud, you're in danger. If your body becomes your identity, you're worshiping the creation instead of the Creator. If you can't rest without guilt, you've made training an idol.

Check your motives regularly. Why do you train? To steward the temple and extend your capacity to serve, or to impress people and feed your ego? The answer reveals whether you're on track or veering into idolatry.

If your training makes you more able to serve, more patient with your family, and more present in ministry, you're on track. If it isolates you, makes you obsessive, or creates pride, you've crossed the line.

PRACTICE PROMPT

- ❖ Consider the warnings from this section, and decide which one resonates the most with you right now.

- ❖ Write one specific way it applies to your current situation.

- ❖ Write one specific action you'll take this week to address it.

Success Criteria

☐ You identified the warning that actually describes you (not the one you *wish* applied).

☐ You wrote a specific current example showing how it's playing out in your life.

☐ You chose one concrete action to address it.

☐ You shared your response with your accountability partner or mentor within forty-eight hours with a request for them to check in next week.

Troubleshooting

If no warning resonated with you, then you're either in excellent health across all areas, or you're blind to your patterns. Ask someone close to you which warning they see in your life. Their answer matters more than yours.

If you identified the warning but didn't share it with someone, you're keeping yourself unaccountable.

If you shared it, but your accountability partner didn't actually check in, you picked someone who won't challenge you. Find someone who will.

THE BODY SERVING THE MISSION

The question isn't whether to train your body. The question is whether you want to serve for thirty years or three, whether you'll be present when your grandkids need you, or whether preventable decline will sideline you early.

Physical training powers everything else. A trained body stabilizes emotions because your nervous system learns to handle stress without breaking down. Chronic cortisol elevation from a sedentary, neglected body destabilizes emotions and shortens your fuse. But when you train consistently, your body learns to activate under pressure and recover afterward.

That regulation doesn't stay in the gym. It shows up when your kid has a meltdown, when work gets chaotic, when relationships hit friction. The heart steadies because the body knows how to process activation instead of drowning in it.

Exercise also triggers BDNF production in the brain, strengthening neural connections and supporting cognitive plasticity. Blood flow improves. Metabolic waste clears faster.

Inflammation drops. The result is sharper thinking during long meetings, faster learning when acquiring new skills, and sustained focus when decisions matter most. A strong body feeds mental clarity because the brain runs on what the body provides. Spiritual disciplines demand endurance. Prayer requires sustained attention. Service requires physical presence over years, not just months.

A weak body gives out early. A trained body sustains the work. The discipline you build physically, the ability to override the voice that says, "quit early," that reflex transfers everywhere. It shows up in your prayer life, in your marriage, in your ministry. Physical discipline teaches spiritual discipline. They're not separate categories. They're integrated.

Your body determines how long you can show up. Strength extends your runway for service. Cardiovascular health keeps you present when others burn out. Mobility prevents the breakdown that sidelines people in their fifties and sixties. Temple maintenance isn't optional if you want to serve well into old age.

Your body is a tool for holiness, not a distraction from it. Steward the temple. Build discipline in the body so the soul can do what it was made to do.

Start simple. Stay consistent. Treat physical care as vocational practice that powers everything else you want to steward well.

This takes years, not weeks. But every session compound

CHAPTER FOUR
A STRONG AND HEALTHY SOUL

"He restores my soul. He leads me in paths of righteousness for his name's sake"

(Psalm 23:3).

UNDERSTANDING A STRONG AND HEALTHY SOUL

The studio was growing. After years of grinding, pivoting, rebuilding, learning, the business was gaining traction. Clients were showing up. Revenue was climbing. People were getting results. From the outside, it looked like everything I'd worked for was coming together.

But then the friction and resistance felt sharper, more pronounced, even. Random people I barely knew started telling me I was on the wrong path. "Are you sure this is what you're supposed to be doing?" they'd ask, unprompted.

I'd brush it off at first, but the frequency was unsettling. Then my body started breaking down. Sickness I couldn't shake. Internal issues that stemmed from the past. I was exhausted in a way that sleep didn't fix.

The pressure mounted. Stress piled on stress. I started questioning everything. *Am I in the right position? Did I miss something? Have I lost my purpose?*

The doubt was suffocating.

But I was still moving. I was pouring into my clients. I was going to church. I was praying. I was doing all the things I thought I was supposed to do. I wasn't skipping spiritual disciplines. I wasn't neglecting my work. From the outside, I was maintaining.

Yet something was deeply wrong.

I couldn't shake the feeling that I was spiritually out of position. Like I was standing in the right place but facing the wrong direction. Or maybe I was in the wrong place entirely. I didn't know. The confusion itself was disorienting.

Finally, I went to my pastor. I laid it all out: the attacks, the sickness, the doubt, the pressure. I told him I was doing everything I knew to do—working, serving, praying, showing up. "So what's wrong," I asked. "What am I missing?"

He listened. Then he said something that shifted everything.

"It sounds like you're doing everything right," he said. "But what's being required of you right now is *more*. You need to make praying and fasting your business."

Not just a practice. *Your business.* The thing you organize your life around. The thing that gets priority, resources, and sustained attention.

I can't say I came through all of it. That season led directly into my father passing away. And even now, as I write this chapter, things are still coming down hard. The attacks haven't stopped. The pressure hasn't lifted. I'm not writing from the other side of this with all the answers tied up neatly.

But I've learned something critical: doing spiritual things is not the same as tending your soul. You can pray without depth. You can read Scripture without absorption. You can attend church without connection. You can maintain all the external disciplines while your soul slowly starves.

Tending of the Life

A strong and healthy soul is the conscious, disciplined tending of the life God breathed into you. Everything else in this chapter builds from that foundation.

There's an urgency to what I'm writing here. I need to get this out to you because I know some of you are where I was:

doing all the right things, wondering why nothing's working, feeling spiritually out of position despite showing up faithfully. You need to know what I'm learning in real time, in the middle of the fire.

The soul isn't maintained through religious routine. It's strengthened through deliberate, sustained, focused engagement with God. And when the pressure rises, when the attacks intensify, when everything feels like it's falling apart despite your faithfulness, the depth of your soul determines whether you stand or collapse.

What follows isn't theory. It's what I'm living. It's what's keeping me upright when everything in me wants to quit. It's the framework that's sustaining me through the hardest season of my life.

You need it. I need it. Let's build it together.

The soul organizes your entire being, where purpose, conscience, and longing converge. When it is watered and tended, your mind thinks clearer, your emotions stabilize, and your body moves with intention. A neglected soul produces brittle thinking, reactive emotions, and inconsistent action. A restored soul creates steady motives, durable habits, and sustainable service.

Psalm 1:2–3 builds the picture:

"His delight is in the law of the Lord, and on his law he meditates day and night. He is like a tree planted by streams of water that yields its fruit in its season" *(Psalm 1:2–3).*

Tending your soul means regulating what enters and what feeds it. It means naming spiritual neglect before it corrodes, refusing laziness before it takes root, and keeping the interior life aligned with truth. Spiritual fitness is how you tend the soul so that what flows out (words, choices, service) carries life instead of decay.

The Language of Restoration and Soundness

Psalm 23:3 gives us the central image:

"He restores my soul. He leads me in paths of righteousness

for his name's sake" (Psalm 23:3).

The Hebrew verb *shub* (restore) sits at the center of this promise. It means to return something to its original state, to bring back what was lost or broken. But *shub* never stands alone in Scripture's vocabulary of wholeness. It works in concert with *rapha*—to heal, to cure, to make whole again. God restores by healing. The two actions are inseparable.

When God completes this work of restoration and healing, the result is *marpeh*—a word carrying the full weight of health, soundness, and wholeness. Not merely the absence of disease, but the presence of vitality. A soul marked by *marpeh* operates with the integrity God intended when He first breathed life into dust.

This same concept appears in Greek. Paul writes of *sōphronismos* in 2 Timothy 1:7—a sound mind, a mental wholeness where thinking, emotion, and will cooperate instead of war against each other. The mind operating with the clarity and discipline God designed.

Sound heart. Sound mind. Strong body. Strong soul.

These aren't arbitrary descriptors. They echo Scripture's understanding that God's work in us produces wholeness. A sound soul is one God has restored through His healing touch, maintained through spiritual disciplines, and strengthened through consistent practice. Scripture applies this same language of restoration and soundness across every dimension of human existence—soul, mind, heart, and body. When God restores, he makes whole.

Here's what this means practically: your soul's condition determines your capacity. When God's restorative work keeps your soul whole and healthy, your thinking sharpens, your emotions stabilize, your body responds with energy instead of exhaustion. But when spiritual neglect sets in, the deterioration spreads. Judgment clouds. Emotions react. The physical breaks down. The soul's health radiates outward, touching every dimension of your existence.

Soundness isn't accidental. It comes through God's intervention meeting your participation. He does the healing work. You show up for the practices that position you to receive it.

How This Connects to the Rest of The SCAL Method

The soul isn't just one more arena to manage. What happens here determines what's possible everywhere else. Unchecked spiritual neglect breeds emotional chaos, but train the soul, and the heart finds its pattern. A depleted soul produces clouded judgment, while spiritual practices require the cognitive discipline that sharpens the mind. Chronic spiritual emptiness wrecks sleep, immunity, and recovery. A restored soul stabilizes the whole person.

You've seen what the soul is and why it matters. Now you need to see what Scripture says about its nature, purpose, and design. The Bible doesn't treat the soul as abstract theology. It treats it as the core of human existence, breathed into being by God Himself.

BIBLICAL FOUNDATION

Genesis 2:7 establishes the foundation:

"Then the Lord God formed the man of dust from the ground and breathed into his nostrils the breath of life, and the man became a living creature" (Genesis 2:7).

The text names the action directly: God formed, God breathed, and the man became alive. The Hebrew word for "living creature" (*nephesh chayyah*) is often translated as "living soul." The breathed life of God is personal, intentional, and crafted. The imagery is intimate: God's breath entering human form, animating dust into life.

Scripture ties the unseen interior to the visible exterior, showing that what rules the soul eventually shows up in the body, the mind, and the actions. This is why physical symptoms and relational breakdowns so often point back to spiritual neglect

Identity and Worth

"For you formed my inward parts; you knitted me

together in my mother's womb. I praise you, for I am fearfully and wonderfully made" (Psalm 139:13–15).

The language here is one of careful workmanship. "Knitted together" speaks to intentional design. This anchors worth and purpose in God's craftsmanship rather than human performance. Your soul (your essential being) is created with purpose. You cultivate what is already made. You don't manufacture identity from insecurity.

"Before I formed you in the womb I knew you, and before you were born I consecrated you" (Jeremiah 1:5).

Identity is given. Calling is appointed. This changes how we approach spiritual growth: we are not creating ourselves from scratch; we are tending what God has already planted.

Scripture as Nourishment

"All Scripture is breathed out by God and profitable for teaching, for reproof, for correction, and for training in righteousness, that the man of God may be complete, equipped for every good work" (2 Timothy 3:16–17).

Scripture is the training manual, the fuel, the corrective lens. It instructs, reproves, corrects, and equips. The Greek word for "breathed out" (*theopneustos*) literally means "God-breathed." The same divine breath that created the soul now speaks through the text to form and restore it. Reading Scripture is how the soul is trained, corrected, and equipped for service.

Restoration and Rest

Psalm 23:2–3 is familiar to many:

"He makes me lie down in green pastures. He leads me beside still waters. He restores my soul" (Psalm 23:2–3).

The shepherd creates conditions for rest, nourishment,

and restoration. Green pastures and still waters are necessities for survival and health. The soul requires regular, intentional restoration. Neglect it, and the whole organism suffers. Tend it, and everything follows.

Scripture establishes what the soul is and how God designed it. But understanding design means nothing without knowing how to maintain it. Four ancient practices form the foundation of soul care, tested across centuries and validated by both Scripture and science.

PRACTICE PROMPT

❖ Read Psalm 139: 13–16 slowly, then pause for two minutes of silence.

❖ Read it again slowly, and pause for two minutes again.

❖ For a third time, read it and pause for two minutes.

❖ Write down one phrase that stands out to you.

❖ Ask yourself, "How does this phrase challenge my current view of myself?"

Success Criteria

□ You sat in silence for the full six minutes without checking your phone or filling the quiet with distraction.

Troubleshooting

If sitting still feels impossible, start with thirty seconds of silence after each reading. Build up over time. The discomfort you feel in silence often reveals what your soul is avoiding.

BUILDING A STRONG SOUL

Spiritual strength is built through consistent practice in four areas: Scripture intake, prayer, worship, and fasting. These aren't novel. They're ancient, tested, and effective. Every major Christian tradition recognizes them as foundational.

These practices work together as a system. Scripture shows

you God's character and will. Prayer connects you to His presence. Worship reorients your focus from yourself to Him. Fasting trains your body to submit to your soul and your soul to submit to God.

Scripture intake is how you hear God speak. The words on the page aren't just information. They're formation. When you read Scripture consistently, it shapes how you think, what you value, and how you respond to life. This is the intake valve for truth.

Prayer is how you speak to God. It's conversation, not performance. Honest communication with the one who already knows everything you're trying to hide. Prayer is where relationship happens, where you bring your real self before God and learn to trust him with what you can't control.

Worship is how you recalibrate your attention. It interrupts self-focus and redirects you toward something infinitely larger than your immediate concerns. Both corporate worship (with others) and personal worship (alone with God) are essential. You need both the collective body and the private encounter.

Fasting is how you train submission. When you intentionally abstain from food or other comforts to focus on God, you're teaching your body that your soul is in charge and your soul answers to God. Fasting reveals what controls you and strengthens your capacity to say no to lesser things for the sake of greater things.

Each practice serves a specific function. Together, they create a complete system for soul health. In the sections that follow, you'll see how each one works and why it matters.

These practices aren't just spiritual exercises. They're biological interventions with measurable effects on your brain and body. Modern neuroscience confirms what Scripture has proclaimed for millennia.

SCIENCE BEHIND SOUL HEALTH

Spiritual practices physically change your brain and body. This isn't metaphor. It's measurable biology.

Meditation and prayer restructure the brain. Research using fMRI imaging shows that consistent meditation and contemplative prayer increase gray matter density in the prefrontal cortex (decision-making, self-control) and hippocampus (memory, learning) while decreasing activity in the amygdala (fear, stress response). Regular practitioners show stronger neural connections in areas responsible for attention, emotional regulation, and empathy.

Translation: Daily spiritual practices don't just make you feel peaceful. They literally rebuild your brain's capacity for focus, emotional stability, and rational decision-making.

Prayer reduces stress hormones. Studies measuring cortisol levels (the primary stress hormone) before and after prayer sessions show significant reductions. Heart rate variability improves, blood pressure stabilizes, and inflammatory markers decrease. The physiological stress response literally calms when the soul engages with God.

Community and belonging extend life. Longitudinal studies tracking thousands of participants over decades show that people with strong spiritual community connections live longer, recover from illness faster, and report higher life satisfaction. Social isolation correlates with increased mortality risk comparable to smoking fifteen cigarettes per day. Spiritual community isn't a nice-to-have. It's a survival factor.

Fasting triggers cellular repair. Research on intermittent shows it activates autophagy (cellular cleanup), reduces oxidative stress, improves insulin sensitivity, and promotes neurogenesis. Biblical fasting isn't just spiritual discipline. It's a biological reset button that enhances brain function and metabolic health.

You've seen what the practices are and what they do to your brain and body. Now it's time to see how each one actually works in practice, starting with the foundation: Scripture intake.

PRACTICE PROMPT

- ❖ Write the date of the last time you felt spiritually alive.

- ❖ Then write one sentence describing what your soul feels like right now. Don't sanitize it. Write what's actually true.

If you can't do this exercise, ask yourself why. That hesitation is data.

- ❖ Text your sentence to one person who knows you well. No explanation is needed. Just send it. Their response will tell you whether you're being honest or performing.

Success Criteria

☐ You actually sent the text within twenty-four hours; you didn't just think about it.

Troubleshooting

If you can't bring yourself to send it, that resistance is telling you something. The soul work you need most is often the work you're avoiding.

PRACTICE ONE: SCRIPTURE INTAKE

Scripture is how God speaks. Reading it is how you listen. This isn't about information transfer. It's about formation. The text shapes how you think, what you value, and how you respond to life.

In 2 Timothy 3:16–17, it says Scripture is "profitable for teaching, for reproof, for correction, and for training in righteousness." Notice the progression: teaching (knowledge), reproof (conviction), correction (change), training (formation). This is a developmental process. You don't read Scripture once and arrive. You read it repeatedly, letting it work on you over time.

The Minimum Effective Dose

Take fifteen minutes daily to do this. That doesn't mean listening to it while driving, or skimming while distracted. It means focused, attentive reading.

This isn't much, but it's enough to create momentum. Most people fail because they aim for an hour and quit after three days. Start with fifteen minutes. Do it consistently. Build from there.

The Method

Pick a book of the Bible. Read it straight through, one chapter per sitting. Don't jump around. Don't cherry-pick favorite passages. Read sequentially.

Read slowly. Let the words land. When you rush, you miss everything. The goal isn't coverage. The goal is comprehension and absorption.

Pause when something strikes you. Write it down. Ask, "What is God saying here? How does this apply to me today?"

If you finish your 15 minutes and can't summarize what you just read, you weren't paying attention. Slow down.

Common Failure Points

Treating it Like a Checkbox

You can read Scripture mechanically and miss everything. If you're just trying to hit your daily reading goal without actually engaging the text, you're wasting time.

Reading Without Retention

If you can't summarize what you just read, slow down. Read less. Absorb more.

Avoiding books that make you uncomfortable. The passages you resist often hold what you need most. Don't skip the hard books. Leviticus, Lamentations, Revelation—read them. They're there for a reason.

What to Expect

The first week feels awkward. You're building a new habit. Your mind will wander. Your phone will call. Push through.

The second week gets easier. The pattern starts to click. You'll notice thoughts from Scripture surfacing during the day.

By week four, skipping feels wrong. The practice has momentum. You're not just reading. You're listening.

Scripture is how you hear God. Prayer is how you respond. Reading without praying is like listening to someone talk and never answering. The conversation is incomplete.

PRACTICE PROMPT

❖ This week, read one chapter per day from the book of James. Set a timer for fifteen minutes. Read slowly.

❖ When the timer goes off, write one sentence summarizing what you read and one sentence about how it applies to you.

Success Criteria

☐ You completed five out of seven days.
☐ You wrote actual summaries and not vague generalizations.

Troubleshooting

If your mind wandered constantly, that's normal. Bring it back each time. If you couldn't write summaries, read slower tomorrow.

PRACTICE TWO: PRAYER

Prayer is conversation with God. It's not performance. It's not eloquence. It's honest communication with the One who already knows everything you're trying to hide.

"Pray without ceasing," we see in 1 Thessalonians 5:17. This doesn't mean constant verbalization. It means living with an ongoing awareness of dependence and connection throughout the day. Brief prayers woven into the fabric of daily life, plus focused prayer time set aside specifically for God.

The Minimum Effective Dose

Ten minutes of focused prayer daily, plus brief prayers throughout the day constitute a minimum effective dose.

Ten minutes feels long when you start. That's the point. You're learning to be still before God, to sit in His presence without rushing to the next thing.

The Method

Start with gratitude. Name three specific things you're thankful for. Not generic platitudes. Specific realities. This reorients your attention toward what God has already done.

Confess. Name sin clearly. Don't soften it. Don't rationalize it. Call it what it is. Confession isn't about feeling bad. It's about staying honest with God and yourself.

Ask. Be specific. God can handle your real requests. Don't sanitize your prayers with religious language. Tell Him what you actually want, what you actually fear, what you actually need.

Listen. Spend time in silence. Let God speak. This is the hardest part. We're trained to fill silence with noise. Resist that impulse. Sit quietly. Wait.

Types of Prayer

Prayer isn't one-dimensional. Scripture models different kinds of prayer for different purposes. Understanding these types expands your capacity to engage with God.

Adoration: This is prayer that focuses entirely on who God is, not what He does. You worship His character, His attributes, His nature. "God, You are holy. You are faithful. You are sovereign." This isn't asking for anything. It's simply magnifying His worth.

Thanksgiving: Different from adoration, thanksgiving focuses on what God has done. Specific acts of provision, protection, guidance, or grace. "Thank You for healing my son. Thank You for the job. Thank You for sustaining me through that season." Gratitude anchors you in reality.

Confession: Honest acknowledgment of sin. Not vague "forgive me for being a sinner" prayers, but specific naming of specific failures. "I lied to my wife. I was selfish with my time. I harbored bitterness toward that person." Confession keeps you honest before God.

Supplication: This is the type of prayer where you bring your needs, desires, and requests to God. "Provide for this financial need. Heal this relationship. Give me wisdom for this decision."

God invites you to ask. Don't spiritualize away your real needs.

Intercession: Praying for others is called intercessory prayer. It's also called standing in the gap for people who need God's intervention. "Protect my children. Strengthen my friend going through loss. Convict that person of their sin." Intercession is love expressed through prayer.

Lament: This is honest grief brought before God. This is the prayer of Job, David, Jeremiah. "Where are You in this? Why is this happening? How long will this last?" Lament isn't doubt. It's trust expressed through raw honesty. God can handle your questions.

Contemplative/Listening Prayer: This is prayer where you speak less and listen more. You sit in silence, waiting for God to speak through impressions, Scripture, clarity, or conviction. This requires the most discipline because silence is uncomfortable.

You don't need to cycle through all seven types every day. But rotating through them prevents prayer from becoming one-note. Some days require lament. Some days call for intercession. Some days need extended adoration. Let your soul's condition and life's circumstances guide which type of prayer you need.

Common Failure Points

Treating Prayer Like a Wish List

Prayer is relationship, not transaction. If every prayer is a request and you never listen, you're not praying. You're placing orders.

Praying Only in Crisis

If you only talk to God when things fall apart, you're training yourself to view Him as emergency services. Prayer is for all of life, not just disasters.

Avoiding Silence

If you can't sit quietly before God for 60 seconds, ask yourself why. What are you avoiding in the silence?

Praying the Same Words Repeatedly

If your prayers sound identical every day, be careful. There's a good chance you are not engaging. We are going for the kind of prayer that responds to real life. Your conversations with God should reflect what's actually happening in your soul.

What to Expect

The first few days, your mind will race. You'll think of forty-seven things you need to do. Let those thoughts pass. Come back to God.

By week two, the silence will feel less oppressive. You'll start to notice God speaking through impressions, Scripture that surfaces, quiet clarity about decisions.

By week four, prayer becomes conversation. Not one-sided performance, but actual back-and-forth with God. You speak. You listen. You notice His responses.

Prayer happens alone with God. But you weren't designed to stay alone. Worship brings you into the collective body, where individual faith is strengthened by communal focus.

PRACTICE PROMPT

* ❖ This week, spend ten minutes in focused prayer each morning. Use the structure: gratitude (three items), confession (one or two specific sins), requests (a few specific asks), silence (two or three minutes of listening).

* ❖ Additionally, practice one different type of prayer each day beyond your morning routine:

  * Day One: Adoration (Focus entirely on God's character.)
  * Day Two: Thanksgiving (List specific things God has done.)
  * Day Three: Intercession (Pray for three specific people by name.)
  * Day Four: Lament (Bring honest grief or questions to God.)
  * Day Five: Supplication (Ask for specific needs to be met.)
  * Day Six: Contemplative prayer (Sit for ten minutes of silence, listening.)
  * Day Seven: Your choice (Use the type you need most

today.)

Success Criteria

☐ You completed five out of seven days.
☐ You actually sat in silence for the full listening period.
☐ You practiced at least four different types of prayer.

Troubleshooting

If you struggled with silence, start with thirty seconds. Build up gradually. The discomfort is normal.

If certain types of prayer feel impossible (especially lament or adoration), that reveals what your soul needs most. Don't avoid it. Press into it.

PRACTICE THREE: WORSHIP

Worship reorients your attention toward God's character and worth. It interrupts self-focus and redirects you toward something infinitely larger than your immediate concerns.

"Let us consider how to stir up one another to love and good works, not neglecting to meet together, as is the habit of some, but encouraging one another"(Hebrews 10:24–25).

Corporate worship isn't optional. It's commanded. You need the collective body to stay calibrated. Isolated Christianity is compromised Christianity. When you worship alone, you lack correction. When you worship together, the body keeps you honest.

The Minimum Effective Dose

Weekly corporate worship plus five minutes of personal worship daily is the minimum effective dose.

Corporate worship means showing up to a local church consistently. Not streaming a service from your couch. Not church-hopping for the best experience. Committed presence in one congregation.

Personal worship means five minutes alone with God, focusing on His character through song, Scripture, or silence. This isn't elaborate. Play one worship song. Sing along. Let the words sink in.

The Method

Corporate worship: Commit to a local church. Show up consistently. Same place, same people, week after week.

Participate fully. Sing even if you don't feel like it. Listen even when distracted. Worship isn't about your emotional state. It's about redirecting your attention toward God regardless of how you feel.

Don't consume worship. Contribute to it. Show up early. Greet people. Serve in some capacity. You're not an audience member. You're part of the body.

Personal worship: Pick one song each morning. Play it while you make coffee or get ready. Sing along. Focus on the words. Let them reorient your mind before the day starts.

If you can't sing, read a Psalm aloud. Psalm 103, 145, or 150 work well. Speak the words. Let them shape your thoughts.

Common Failure Points

Attending Without Engaging

Presence doesn't equal participation. If you show up physically but check out mentally, you're wasting time.

Church Shopping Indefinitely

There is no perfect church. Pick one that preaches the gospel faithfully, loves people genuinely, and serves the community actively. Then commit. Stay through the hard seasons.

Skipping When Inconvenient

The discipline is the point. When you only show up when it's convenient, you're making worship optional. It's not.

What to Expect

The first few weeks, corporate worship might feel awkward. You're new. People don't know you. The music isn't your style. Push through.

By week four, faces become familiar. You start to recognize people. Conversations happen. You're not just attending. You're joining.

By month three, you're invested. You know names. You serve somewhere. When you miss a Sunday, people notice. You're part of the body.

Worship reorients your attention. Fasting reorients your submission. When you fast, you're training your body to obey your soul and your soul to obey God.

PRACTICE PROMPT

* ❖ This month, attend the same church every Sunday. Arrive ten minutes early. Greet at least two people. Stay ten minutes after the service. Talk to someone.

* ❖ Additionally, play one worship song each morning for five minutes. Sing along or read a Psalm aloud.

Success Criteria

☐ You attended church four out of four Sundays.
☐ You greeted people and stayed after.
☐ You did personal worship twenty or more days.

Troubleshooting

If you're struggling to find a church, visit three or four options, pick one, and commit for ninety days. If you're avoiding people, start with one conversation per week.

PRACTICE FOUR: FASTING

Fasting is the intentional abstaining from food (or other comforts) to focus on God. It trains your body to submit to your will and your will to submit to God's.

"When you fast, do not look gloomy like the hypocrites."
(Matthew 6:16).

Notice the assumption: when you fast, not if you fast. Jesus expected His followers to fast. It's not optional for the spiritually advanced. It's normal practice for all believers.
Medical Note: Consult a doctor before fasting if you have

health conditions, take medications, or have a history of disordered eating. Fasting should strengthen you, not harm you. If you're pregnant, nursing, diabetic, or have other medical concerns, modify or skip this practice with medical guidance.

The Minimum Effective Dose

Do one twenty-four-hour fast per month. This isn't extreme. It's sustainable. From dinner one day to dinner the next day. You skip breakfast and lunch. You drink water. When hunger hits, you pray instead of eating.

The Method

Pick a day each month. Mark it on your calendar. Treat it like any other appointment.

Fast from dinner to dinner. Eat a normal meal the night before. Skip breakfast and lunch the next day. Break the fast with a simple dinner.

When hunger hits (and it will), pray. Use the hunger as a reminder to turn your attention to God. Every time your stomach growls, thank God for something. Pray for someone. Read Scripture.

Break the fast with something simple and nutritious. Don't binge. Don't overeat. Just have a normal meal.

Common Failure Points

Fasting with pride

If you tell everyone you're fasting, check your motives. Jesus warned against public fasting for recognition. Fast quietly. Let God see it. That's enough.

Fasting Without Prayer

Hunger alone doesn't build spiritual muscle. Fasting without prayer is just skipping meals. The point is to redirect your attention from food to God.

Ignoring Genuine Health Contraindications

If your doctor says don't fast, then don't fast. Fasting should serve your stewardship, not undermine it. There's no spiritual points for hurting yourself.

What to Expect

The first few hours are easy. You're not that hungry yet.

Hours six through twelve are hard. Your body wants food. Your mind invents reasons to quit. Push through.

Hours eighteen through twenty-four often bring clarity. The hunger levels out. Your mind feels sharper. You notice dependence you usually ignore.

When you break the fast, food tastes better. You're more aware of provision. You've practiced submission and come out stronger.

You've seen each practice individually: Scripture, prayer, worship, fasting. But they don't function in isolation. They work together as a complete system. The framework shows you how.

PRACTICE PROMPT

❖ This month, schedule one full-day fast. Pick a day. Mark your calendar. Fast from dinner to dinner.

❖ When hunger hits, pray for two minutes. Thank God for provision. Ask him to meet a specific need. Read one Psalm.

Success Criteria

☐ You completed the full twenty-four hours.
☐ You prayed every time hunger hit.
☐ You broke the fast with a normal meal, not a binge.

Troubleshooting

If you failed to complete it, identify why. Was it physical (genuine health issue) or mental (discomfort, inconvenience)? If mental, try again next month. If physical, consult a doctor before trying again.

THE FRAMEWORK

Soul health isn't built through random spiritual activity. It's built through a repeatable cycle that integrates all four practices into one coherent system.

Receive. Reflect. Respond. Repeat.

This is the pattern that builds and maintains spiritual strength.

Receive

Receive truth through Scripture, prayer, worship, and community.

Scripture is the primary input. God speaks through His Word. You receive teaching, correction, instruction, and encouragement. Prayer is two-way conversation. You speak, but you also listen. You receive God's guidance, conviction, comfort, and direction.

Worship is corporate and personal. You receive perspective when you gather with others and when you focus on God alone. Community provides input you can't get solo. You receive correction, encouragement, challenge, and support from other believers who see what you miss.

This is the intake phase. You're filling the tank. You can't give what you haven't received.

Reflect

Reflect on truth via meditation, journaling, and contemplation.

Meditation means thinking deeply about what you've received. It's not emptying your mind but filling it with Scripture and letting it sink in. Chew on truth until it becomes part of you. Journaling means writing what you're learning, feeling, and questioning. The act of writing forces clarity. Vague thoughts become concrete when you put them on paper.

Contemplation means sitting with truth in silence. Let it work on you without rushing to application. Sometimes the most important work happens in stillness.

This is the processing phase. You're letting truth move from your head to your heart.

Respond

Respond to truth through obedience, service, repentance, and witness.

Obedience means doing what God says, not just knowing it. It's also not just agreeing with it. It's actually doing it. Truth that doesn't produce action is worthless.

Service means using your strength for others. A healthy soul overflows into service. If your spiritual practices never result in serving people, something is broken.

Repentance means changing direction when you're wrong: confessing sin, turning from it, and moving toward holiness. This is ongoing, not a one-time thing.

Witness means sharing what God has done—not preaching at people, but testifying to reality. When God changes you, you tell people about it.

This is the output phase. You're living what you've learned.

Repeat

Repeat the pattern through daily, weekly, and monthly practices.

- **Daily:** Fifteen minutes Scripture, ten minutes prayer, five minutes worship, journaling as needed
- **Weekly:** Corporate worship, small group or spiritual friendship, service to church or community
- **Monthly:** Extended prayer/retreat (two to three hours), fasting (twenty-four hours), comprehensive review of progress

This is the sustainability phase. You're building lasting patterns.

How the Framework Functions

The cycle isn't linear. You don't finish one phase to never return. You're always in multiple phases simultaneously.

You receive truth while responding to previous truth. You reflect on yesterday's Scripture while receiving today's input. You serve others while continuing to receive from God.

The framework is a spiral, not a straight line. Each cycle deepens the previous one. You revisit the same truths at different depths. You apply the same principles to new situations.

Over time, the framework becomes automatic. You don't consciously think, *I'm in the receive phase now.* You just live the pattern. Receive, reflect, respond, repeat becomes how you operate.

The framework shows you how soul health is built. But before you can build, you need to assess current condition.

Spiritual decay is insidious because it disguises itself as busyness, productivity, or even ministry. You need to recognize the patterns before the damage compounds.

PRACTICE PROMPT

This week, implement the complete framework daily:

- ❖ **Receive:** Fifteen minutes Scripture, ten minutes of prayer (including listening).
- ❖ **Reflect:** Five minutes journaling what struck you from Scripture or prayer.
- ❖ **Respond:** Identify one specific action from today's input and do it.
- ❖ **Repeat:** Do this sequence six out of seven days.

Success Criteria

☐ You completed the full cycle six days.
☐ You can point to specific actions you took in response to what you received.

Troubleshooting

If you missed days, identify the breakdown point. Was it the receive phase (didn't make time)? Reflect phase (skipped journaling)? Respond phase (didn't act)? Focus on strengthening your weak link.

SPIRITUAL NEGLECT

Spiritual neglect doesn't announce itself. It creeps in through small compromises, justified delays, and rationalized shortcuts. By the time you notice the damage, the corrosion is already deep. The drift follows a predictable pattern. First, you skip one spiritual discipline, just once. You're tired, busy, overwhelmed. It feels reasonable. Then it happens again, and again. The gap between intention and practice widens.

Prayer becomes sporadic. Scripture reading becomes optional. Worship attendance becomes weather-dependent. Community becomes convenient. You tell yourself you'll get back to it when life calms down.

But life doesn't calm down. It intensifies. And without the soul's anchor, you become reactive instead of responsive, anxious instead of steady, and empty instead of full.

Real-World Example: Desmond

When Desmond's patience with his four-year-old son Marcus thinned to nothing, when his shoulders stayed knotted for three weeks straight, when he snapped at his wife Rachel over dishes left in the sink, the problem wasn't time management or personality conflict.

The problem was three levels deeper.

Desmond didn't see it at first. The drift is slow.

Three weeks prior, he stopped his morning Scripture reading. "Too busy," he told himself.

Then he skipped prayer. Then small group. Then it was Sunday worship he missed—once, then twice.

Desmond said, "I'll catch up when things calm down."

Things don't calm down. They compound.

Desmond's anxiety about work climbed. His decisions became shortsighted. He felt spiritually empty but couldn't figure out why. His soul was running on fumes, and the physical evidence was everywhere: the short temper, the chronic tension, the inability to be present with his family.

The soul keeps score. You can ignore the scorecard, but the numbers don't change.

Physical Symptoms of Spiritual Neglect

Your body broadcasts what your soul won't say:

- Chronic fatigue that sleep doesn't fix
- Tension that stretches across your shoulders and refuses to release
- Headaches with no discernable medical cause
- Digestive issues that doctors can't explain

- Insomnia despite exhaustion

These aren't always spiritual problems, but when medical solutions fail and the symptoms persist, the soul may be screaming what you refuse to hear.

The research backs up the possibility of a connection. Studies show that people who regularly engage in spiritual practices report better sleep quality, lower rates of depression and anxiety, improved immune function, and faster recovery from illness. The soul's health directly affects the body's function. Neglect one, and you will damage both.

Emotional and Relational Symptoms

Irritability without clear cause, emotional flatness where joy used to live, cynicism replacing hope, and impatience with people you love are markers of a soul running dry.

Relationships corrode when the soul is neglected. You become transactional instead of relational and keep score instead of offering grace. You withdraw instead of engage. Your capacity for empathy shrinks, and your patience evaporates. The people closest to you feel the distance, even if they can't name it.

Mental and Decision-Making Symptoms

A neglected soul produces clouded thinking. Decisions take longer. Clarity becomes elusive. You second-guess yourself constantly. Priorities blur. What used to feel obvious now feels complicated. You drift toward reactivity instead of intentionality. This happens because spiritual neglect depletes the interior resources that fuel good judgment. Without regular spiritual input, your mental frameworks weaken. You lose the ability to distinguish signal from noise, truth from distraction, wisdom from mere information.

The Progression of Spiritual Decay

Spiritual collapse rarely happens all at once; it unfolds quietly, step by step, long before you realize what you've lost.

Stage One is the slip. You miss one discipline. It feels minor. You justify it.

Stage Two is the pattern. Missing becomes regular. You rationalize it as temporary.

Stage Three is the drift. Weeks pass without engagement. You notice but do nothing.

Stage Four is the emptiness. You feel spiritually dead but can't pinpoint when it started.

Stage Five is the crisis. Something breaks. A relationship, a decision, a moral failure. The foundation wasn't there when you needed it.

Most people don't recognize the pattern until Stage Four or Five. By then, the repair work is extensive. The goal is to catch it at Stage One or Two, before the damage compounds.

You've seen the symptoms. You've named the neglect. Now comes the building phase: creating sustainable structure that makes spiritual practices automatic, not optional.

PRACTICE PROMPT

Answer these diagnostic questions with brutal honesty. Write your answers. Don't just think them.

* When was the last time I read Scripture for more than five minutes?

* When was the last time I prayed beyond a meal blessing or crisis plea?

* When was the last time I worshiped with others?

* When was the last time I had a substantive spiritual conversation?

* What spiritual discipline have I abandoned in the past month? Why?

Success Criteria

☐ You wrote actual answers, not vague approximations.
☐ You named specific dates and specific reasons.

Troubleshooting

If you can't remember dates, that's the answer. The gap is larger than you thought. Don't spiral into shame. Use this data to build a plan.

BUILDING SPIRITUAL STRUCTURE

Discipline without structure collapses. You need systems that make spiritual practices automatic, not optional. The goal is to build a daily pattern where these disciplines become as nonnegotiable as brushing your teeth.

The Forty-Minute Morning Block

Most people fail at spiritual disciplines because they try to fit them into leftover time. There is no leftover time. You must carve it out deliberately.

The Framework

- Fifteen minutes: Scripture
- Ten minutes: Prayer
- Five minutes: Worship
- Ten minutes: Journaling (reflecting on what you read, heard, or sensed)

The Setup

Wake up forty minutes earlier than normal. Yes, this requires sacrifice. Yes, it will be hard at first. Do it anyway.

The Execution

Eliminate decision fatigue. Same time, same place, same sequence every day. Remove distractions. Phone off, door closed, environment controlled. Start immediately. Don't check email first. Don't scroll social media. Go straight into the block.

The Adaptation

If mornings don't work, use your lunch break or evening. The time of day matters less than the consistency.

Example: Desmond's 40-Minute Morning

Desmond set his alarm for 5:30 AM. The first week was brutal. His body screamed for more sleep. His mind invented reasons to skip. But Rachel had noticed the change in him over the previous month, the irritability and distance, and when he told her he was committing to morning spiritual practices, she said, "Good. You need it. We need it."

That accountability mattered.

Week one, he made it four out of seven days. It was not perfect but was progress. He read through James, prayed for his family by name, played one worship song, and journaled three sentences about what struck him.

Week two, he hit five out of seven days. The pattern started clicking. He noticed his patience with Marcus improving. It wasn't dramatically, just small moments. The ability to take a breath before reacting was returning.

Week four, Desmond succeeded on six out of seven days. The practices became automatic. His soul felt less empty—not full yet, but filling. Rachel commented that he seemed more present at dinner, more engaged, and less checked out.

Three months in, the forty-minute block is nonnegotiable. Desmond's relationships are stronger. His decision-making is clearer. His capacity to serve has expanded. The soul keeps score, and consistent deposits compound.

THE WEEKLY SABBATH

Sabbath is the structure that sustains all other structures. It's a full day set aside for rest, worship, and restoration. Without it, you will burn out. This isn't simply time off. It's commanded rest.

What To Do

- Pick one full day per week. Protect it.
- Do no work or errands. Don't worry about productivity.
- Focus on worship, rest, relationships, and joy.
- Let yourself be unproductive. The world won't collapse.

The Common Resistance

"I can't afford a full day off." You can't afford not to. Your output will improve when you rest well. Your relationships will strengthen when you're present. Your soul will stabilize when you stop treating rest as weakness.

The Monthly Retreat

Once per month, take two or three hours for extended time with God. This isn't the daily pattern. This is deeper work.

The Habit

Find a quiet place. Leave your normal environment.

- Bring only your Bible, a journal, and a pen.
- Read extended passages. Pray longer. Sit in silence.
- Review the past month. What worked? What didn't? What needs to change?

Accountability Structures

You will not maintain these patterns alone. You need external accountability.

The Framework

Find one person who will ask you weekly: "Did you do your spiritual practices this week?"

- Share your schedule with them. Give them permission to push you.
- Report honestly. Lying to your accountability partner is worse than skipping the practice.

You can build personal spiritual strength, but you cannot grow alone. The next section addresses the role of community in soul health. This isn't about adding more obligations. It's about recognizing that your spiritual formation is incomplete without others.

PRACTICE PROMPT

Do the following for the next month:

- ❖ Implement the forty-minute morning block (or equivalent time) six days per week.
- ❖ Observe a full Sabbath day once per week.

❖ Schedule one monthly retreat (two to three hours).

❖ Find one accountability partner and report to them weekly.

Success Criteria

☐ You completed eighty percent of your intended practices.
☐ You met with your accountability partner at least three times.

Troubleshooting

If you failed this, don't restart. Keep going from where you are. Missing a week doesn't erase the previous work. Guilt doesn't build discipline. Persistence does.

SPIRITUAL COMMUNITY

Christianity is not a solo endeavor. You were designed to grow in the context of community. Isolated faith becomes distorted faith. You need other believers to sharpen you, correct you, encourage you, and call out your blind spots.

"Iron sharpens iron, and one man sharpens another" *(Proverbs 27:17).*

The sharpening process is uncomfortable. It involves friction.

But friction is how you get sharp. Comfort is how you stay dull.

Why You Need a Local Church

"Let us consider how to stir up one another to love and good works, not neglecting to meet together, as is the habit of some, but encouraging one another" *(Hebrews 10:24–25).*

The command is clear: continue meeting together. This isn't about attending as a consumer. This is about committing as a member.

You show up. You serve. You give.

Submit to leadership. Invest in relationships, and stay when it's hard. **The failure mode** is church shopping indefinitely. Treating church like a product you sample until you find the perfect fit. There is no perfect church. Pick one that preaches the gospel faithfully, loves people genuinely, and serves the community actively. Then commit.

Small Groups

Weekly corporate worship isn't enough. You need a smaller group where you're known and people see past the Sunday version of you. In a small group, honesty should be expected and superficiality rejected.

Join a small group. If your church doesn't have them, start a group yourself.

Show up consistently. Missing creates gaps in relationship.

Be honest. Perfection isn't the goal; growth is.

Ask hard questions. Challenge each other. Don't settle for safe conversations.

Spiritual Friendship

Beyond the group, you need at least one person who knows you deeply. Choose someone who will ask the questions you don't want to answer. They should call you out when you drift. It needs to be someone who cares more about your spiritual health than your comfort.

Identify one person who takes their faith seriously. Ask them to meet regularly (weekly or every other week). Give them permission to ask about your spiritual practices, your struggles, your sins.

Do the same for them. This is mutual accountability, not one-way supervision.

Serving the Community

Spiritual health isn't self-contained. It overflows into service. If your spiritual practices never result in serving others, something is broken.

Find one consistent way to serve in your church. For example, volunteer in a ministry.

Find one consistent way to serve your neighborhood. Do tangible acts of service.

Serve without recognition. Anonymous service reveals one's true motives.

Practices and community create the environment for growth,

but growth itself shows up as character change. The next section addresses the specific character traits that mark a healthy soul and how to cultivate them.

PRACTICE PROMPT

Do these things over the next ninety days:

- ❖ Commit to a local church, and go weekly.

- ❖ Join (or start) a small group. Attend consistently.

- ❖ Establish one spiritual friendship. Meet at least twice per month.

- ❖ Volunteer in one church ministry and one community service opportunity.

Success Criteria

□ At the end of ninety days, you attended church ten or more times.
□ You attended small group eight or more times.
□ You met with your spiritual friend six or more times.
□ You have served in your church and community at least once each.

Troubleshooting

If you're resisting community, examine why. Is it fear of vulnerability? Pride? Past hurt? Name the obstacle. Then address it. Isolation will destroy you slowly. Community keeps you tethered to reality.

CULTIVATING CHARACTER

Spiritual practices are tools for cultivating spiritual character. The goal is transformation. Specifically, transformation into Christlikeness. The Bible calls this the fruit of the Spirit: observable character traits that begin to emerge and increase when the Spirit works in you.

216

"But the fruit of the Spirit is love, joy, peace, patience, kindness, goodness, faithfulness, gentleness, self-control" (Galatians 5:22–23).

Notice the word *fruit*. You don't manufacture these traits through effort. You cultivate them through cooperation with the Spirit. The practices create conditions. The Spirit produces the fruit.

Love

Love is the foundation. Without it, everything else is noise. Love means willing the good of another, even at cost to yourself. This isn't feeling. This is choice.

The Cultivation

- Serve someone who can't repay you.
- Exhibit patience with someone who frustrates you.
- Be generous with someone who doesn't deserve it.

The Measure

Are you easier to love this year than last? Are your relationships stronger? Do people feel safer around you?

Joy

Joy isn't happiness. Happiness depends on circumstances. Joy is steady contentment rooted in God's character, regardless of circumstances.

The Cultivation

Express gratitude daily. Name three specific things for which you are thankful.

- Worship when you don't feel like it. Joy often follows obedience instead of preceding it.
- Celebrate others' wins without comparison or envy.

The Measure

Can you experience peace in chaos? Do you celebrate when

nothing is going well? Can you find God's goodness in hard seasons?

Peace

Peace is interior calm when external circumstances warrant panic. It's trusting God's sovereignty when nothing makes sense.

The Cultivation

Pray instead of worrying. When anxiety rises, pray specifically about what's triggering it.

- Let go. Not everything requires your intervention.
- Be silent. Constant noise breeds constant agitation.

The Measure

How quickly do you spiral into anxiety? How long does it take you to recalibrate? Are you becoming steadier over time?

Patience

Patience is the ability to endure delay, frustration, or suffering without collapsing into anger or despair.

The Cultivation

Take a 10-second pause before responding when triggered.

- Wait without complaining. Traffic, lines, delays become training grounds.
- Extend grace to people who test you repeatedly.

The Measure

Are you quicker to anger this year than last? Do small frustrations derail you? Can you endure hardship without bitterness?

More Fruit of the Spirit

The traits of kindness, goodness, faithfulness, gentleness, and self-control cluster together. Kindness is active compassion. Goodness is moral integrity. Faithfulness is reliability. Gentleness is strength under control. Self-control is mastery over impulses.

- Kindness: Do one unexpected act of service daily.
- Goodness: Do the right thing when no one is watching.
- Faithfulness: Keep your word, even when it costs you.
- Gentleness: Respond softly when provoked.
- Self-control: Daily, say no to one thing you want (not need).

The Measure

Are you becoming more like Christ? Not in vague aspiration, but in concrete behavior? Do the people closest to you see the change?

Growing spiritual character sounds peaceful. It's not. You have an enemy who wants you weak, distracted, and defeated.

The next section addresses spiritual warfare: the reality of opposition and how to fight well.

PRACTICE PROMPT

- ❖ Be honest with yourself, and pick your weakest fruit of the Spirit.

- ❖ For the next month, focus specifically on cultivating that one trait.

Here's an example: "Patience is my weakest fruit. This month, I will practice the ten-second pause before responding when triggered. I will pray for patience every morning. I will ask my spouse to tell me when I'm being impatient."

Success Criteria

☐ At the end of thirty days, you can point to specific instances where you practiced this fruit.

☐ You improved, even if not perfectly.

Troubleshooting

If you see no change, you're probably not being specific enough. Generalized effort produces generalized results. Pick one concrete behavior. Practice it repeatedly.

SPIRITUAL WARFARE

If you take your spiritual health seriously, you will face resistance. Some of it will come from within (laziness, doubt, distraction). Some of it will come from without (spiritual opposition).

"For we do not wrestle against flesh and blood but against the rulers, against the authorities, against the cosmic powers over this present darkness, against the spiritual forces of evil in the heavenly places" (Ephesians 6:12).

This isn't a metaphor. There are spiritual forces that actively oppose your growth. Recognizing this reality doesn't mean being paranoid. It means becoming prepared.

Internal Resistance: The Flesh

Your sinful nature resists holiness. It wants comfort, not discipline. It wants pleasure, not obedience. It wants ease, not growth.

The Pattern

- You commit to spiritual practices.
- You start strong.
- The novelty fades.
- The resistance increases.
- You rationalize quitting.

The Counter

Expect the resistance. It's not a sign you're doing it wrong. It's a sign you're doing it right.

- Push through the dip. The breakthrough comes after the resistance, not before.
- Don't rely on feelings. Do the practice whether you feel like it or not.

External Resistance: The Enemy

Satan's strategy is simple: distract, discourage, and destroy. He doesn't need you to renounce faith. He just needs you to neglect your soul long enough that you become ineffective. Below are listed the tactics and how to counter them.

The Tactics

- Distraction: Keeping you busy with good things so you miss the best things
- Discouragement: Convincing you that effort is futile and change is impossible
- Accusation: Reminding you of past failures to paralyze future action

The Counter

- Guard your attention. What you focus on shapes you.
- Remember your identity. You are a child of God, not your worst moment.
- Fight with truth. The enemy lies. Scripture tells the truth.

The Armor of God

Ephesians 6:13–17 describes the armor: truth, righteousness, the gospel, faith, salvation, and the word of God. These aren't metaphorical suggestions. They're actual defenses.

- Truth: Reject lies about God, yourself, and others.
- Righteousness: Live with integrity even when it costs you.
- Gospel: Remember that you're saved by grace, not performance.
- Faith: Trust God when circumstances contradict his promises.
- Salvation: Rest in your secure position in Christ.
- Word of God: Use Scripture to counter lies and temptation.

The Power of Prayer in Warfare

Prayer isn't passive. It's active engagement with God against spiritual opposition. When you pray, you're not hoping God might help. You're partnering with Him in the work He's already doing.

Pray specifically against spiritual attacks. Name them. Ask for protection over your mind, your relationships, and your practices. Pray for discernment to recognize lies and deception

Fighting well requires preparation and practice. But sometimes the fight isn't loud. Sometimes it's silent. When God feels distant despite your faithfulness, when the practices feel mechanical and the breakthrough seems impossible, you need a different kind of endurance.

PRACTICE PROMPT

Whenever you face resistance to spiritual practices, do the following:

- ❖ Pause and ask: Is this internal (flesh) or external (enemy)?

- ❖ If it's internal, push through with discipline. Don't negotiate.

- ❖ If it's external, pray immediately. Name the opposition. Ask God for strength.

- ❖ Do the practice anyway. Resistance doesn't get a vote.

Success Criteria

☐ You recognize resistance as normal, not exceptional.
☐ You fight it instead of surrendering to it.

Troubleshooting

If you're constantly losing the fight, check your supports. Are you isolated? Are you neglecting Scripture? Are you skipping prayer? Warfare requires readiness. It's better to build the armor before the battle, not during it.

WHEN THINGS GET SILENT

There will be seasons when you do everything right and feel nothing. You read Scripture faithfully, but the words seem flat. You pray consistently, but heaven feels like concrete. You worship regularly, but joy is absent. You fast and wait, and the waiting stretches longer than you thought possible.

This is spiritual dryness. The dark night of the soul. The wilderness between promise and fulfillment.

This is normal. This is not failure.

The Reality of Spiritual Dryness

Spiritual dryness doesn't mean you've done something wrong. Sometimes it means you're doing everything right, and God is testing the depth of your commitment. Will you serve Him for what He gives, or for who He is?

Job experienced this. He lost everything. His friends accused him. God seemed silent. But Job's response reveals the conviction that endures dryness:

"Though he slay me, I will hope in him" (Job 13:15).

David experienced this. Psalm 13:1–2 captures his anguish: *"How long, O Lord? Will you forget me forever? How long will you hide your face from me? How long must I take counsel in my soul and have sorrow in my heart all the day?"* (Psalm 13:1–2).

Even Jesus experienced this. On the cross, he cried out: *"My God, my God, why have you forsaken me?"* (Matthew 27:46).

If these men experienced seasons of silence, you will, too. The question is not whether dryness will come. The question is what you do when it arrives.

What Spiritual Dryness Is Not

Spiritual dryness is not the same as spiritual neglect. Neglect is chosen. Dryness is imposed. Neglect comes from laziness.

Dryness comes despite discipline.

Dryness is not the same as depression. Depression is a medical condition that may require professional treatment. Dryness is a spiritual season that requires faithful endurance. They can overlap, but they're not identical.

If you're experiencing prolonged hopelessness, inability to function, or thoughts of self-harm, seek professional help immediately.

Dryness is not punishment. God is not withholding His presence because you've failed. Sometimes He withdraws the feeling of His presence to deepen your faith.

Feeling is not the same as reality. God's presence doesn't depend on your perception.

How to Endure Spiritual Dryness

Keep doing the practices. This is the most important instruction. When you feel nothing, do the disciplines anyway. Read Scripture even when it feels dry. Pray even when heaven seems silent. Worship even when joy is absent. The practices sustain you when feelings fail.

The temptation in dryness is to quit. "If God isn't showing up, why bother?" This is the exact moment to press in harder. Feelings follow faithfulness, not the other way around.

Trust God's character, not your circumstances. God's faithfulness doesn't change based on how you feel. He is the same yesterday, today, and forever (Hebrews 13:8). Your emotions are variable. His nature is constant.

When you can't sense His presence, remember His promises. When you can't feel His love, rehearse His actions. He sent His Son. He paid your debt. He seated you with Christ. These are facts, not feelings.

Look for God in unexpected places. Sometimes God speaks through silence. Sometimes He works through absence. Sometimes the wilderness is where He does His deepest formation.

In dryness, you learn to trust God for who He is, not for what He provides. You learn to serve Him without the reward of good feelings. You learn that faithfulness isn't contingent on emotional payoff.

Talk to someone who's been through it. Dryness feels isolating, but it's common. Find someone who's weathered spiritual dryness and ask them how they endured. Their testimony will remind you that this season ends.

Don't make major decisions in dryness. When you're spiritually dry, everything looks bleak. Your judgment is clouded. Don't quit your church. Don't abandon your calling. Don't make permanent decisions based on temporary feelings.

Watch for the subtle shift. Dryness doesn't usually end dramatically. It fades gradually. One day, you'll realize the heaviness has lifted. The words of Scripture will strike deeper. Prayer will feel less like shouting into a void. Joy will return, quieter than before but more durable.

What Dryness Produces

Seasons of dryness are not wasted. They produce endurance. These times will separate shallow faith from deep roots. They reveal whether you're serving God for his gifts or for himself.

After dryness, your faith is less dependent on feelings. Your worship is more honest. Your prayers are less performative. You've learned to trust God when you can't trace him.

The wilderness is where Moses met God at the burning bush. The desert is where John the Baptist prepared the way. The forty days of fasting is where Jesus faced temptation and emerged victorious.

Dryness is not the end of your story. It's often the beginning of something deeper.

Whether you're experiencing abundance or dryness, the practices remain the same.

The next section shows you how to build spiritual practices into automatic habits so they don't require constant willpower.

PRACTICE PROMPT

If you're in a season of spiritual dryness, do these things:

- ❖ Commit to continuing your spiritual practices for thirty more days, regardless of how you feel.

- ❖ Write down three truths about God's character that don't depend on your current emotional state.

❖ Find one person who's experienced spiritual dryness and ask them, "How did you endure it?"

❖ Read through the Psalms, and highlight every passage where the psalmist expresses feeling distant from God, then note how the Psalm resolves.

Success Criteria

☐ You faithfully completed thirty days despite feeling nothing.
☐ You talked to one person about their experience.

Troubleshooting

If the dryness persists beyond several months and is accompanied by inability to function, seek professional help. Spiritual dryness and clinical depression can overlap, and there's no shame in getting support for either.

SPIRITUAL AUTOMATION

Willpower is finite. Habits are automatic. The goal is to move spiritual practices from conscious effort to unconscious routine. You want these disciplines to become so ingrained that skipping them feels wrong.

The Habit Loop of Cue, Routine, Reward

Every habit follows a pattern:

- Cue: The trigger that initiates the behavior
- Routine: The behavior itself
- Reward: The benefit that reinforces the behavior

The Application

- Cue: Wake up (immediate trigger for morning spiritual practices)
- Routine: 40-minute morning block (Scripture, prayer, worship, journaling)

- Reward: Mental clarity, spiritual peace, sense of accomplishment

Implementation Intentions

Research shows that people who use "if–then" planning are significantly more likely to follow through on commitments.

The Framework

- "If it's six AM, then I read Scripture for 15 minutes."
- "If I sit down for lunch, then I pray first."
- "If I get in the car, then I turn on worship music."

The specificity removes decision fatigue. You're not deciding whether to do it. You're just executing the plan.

Environment Design

Your environment shapes your behavior more than your intentions do. Design your space to make spiritual practices easier and distractions harder. Here's how:

- Create a dedicated space for your morning practices.
- Keep your Bible in the exact spot where you'll read it.
- Set out your journal the night before.
- Charge your phone in another room so it's not the first thing you reach for.

Tracking and Measurement

What gets measured gets improved. Track your spiritual practices daily.

- Use a simple checklist or habit tracker app.
- Mark each day you complete your practices.
- Review weekly.
- Identify patterns.
- Adjust as needed.

The goal is 80% consistency, not perfection. If you hit six out of seven days, you're winning. If you drop below 80%, something needs to change.

Individual habits are building blocks. But spiritual health requires integration across all four arenas. The next section shows you how soul health connects to heart, mind, and body.

PRACTICE PROMPT

Build one spiritual habit using the full framework:

- ❖ Pick one practice (Scripture, prayer, worship, or fasting).

- ❖ Define your cue (what triggers it).

- ❖ Define your routine (what you'll do).

- ❖ Define your reward (what benefit you'll notice).

- ❖ Design your environment to support it.

- ❖ Track it daily for twenty-one days.

Success Criteria

☐ You completed the practice at least seventeen out of twenty-one days (80% or more).

Troubleshooting

If you failed, examine your cue. Is it consistent? Is it clear? Most habit failures happen because the trigger is vague or inconsistent.

SCAL METHOD INTEGRATION

Your soul doesn't operate in isolation. It affects and is affected by your heart, mind, and body. True fitness requires integration.

Soul and Heart

A strong soul stabilizes emotions. Spiritual practices build interior resources that emotional regulation requires. Prayer teaches patience. Worship reorients perspective. Scripture provides truth when feelings lie.

Conversely, unregulated emotions destabilize the soul. Chronic anger, unchecked anxiety, and unprocessed grief drain spiritual energy. You can't maintain spiritual disciplines when your emotional state is chaotic. Do the following:

- Use prayer to process instead of suppressing emotions.
- Use Scripture to challenge distorted emotional patterns.
- Use worship to shift emotional focus from yourself to God.

Soul and Mind

Spiritual practices require cognitive discipline to be effective. Reading Scripture with comprehension, praying with focus, and meditating with attention all sharpen your mental capacity. The soul trains the mind.

Conversely, a lazy mind undermines spiritual growth. If you can't focus for fifteen minutes, you can't engage Scripture deeply. If you can't think critically, you can't discern truth from error. Integrate it by doing these:

- Treat Scripture reading as intellectual training, not just spiritual input.
- Practice contemplative prayer to build concentration.
- Memorize Scripture to strengthen mental recall and combat cognitive decline.
- Soul and Body

Spiritual practices affect physical health. Prayer reduces cortisol. Fasting triggers autophagy. Community reduces mortality risk. The soul's health shows up in the body's function.

Explicit Connection

Scripture makes this connection explicit. John prayed that his readers would be "in good health, as it goes well with your soul" (3 John 1:2). The soul's condition directly determines the body's capacity. Proverbs declares that God's words are "healing (*marpeh*) to all their flesh" (4:22). The same word for soundness that marks a restored soul now extends to physical restoration. The psalmist celebrates that God "forgives all your iniquity" and "heals all your diseases" in the same breath (Psalm 103:3), linking spiritual restoration with bodily healing.

This isn't a metaphor. When your soul runs on fumes, your body pays the price. Conversely, physical neglect undermines spiritual capacity. Chronic sleep deprivation, poor nutrition, and sedentary living all reduce your ability to sustain spiritual disciplines. You can't pray well when exhausted. You can't focus on Scripture when your blood sugar is crashing.

This is what you can do:

- Use physical discipline (exercise, sleep, nutrition) to support spiritual practices.
- Use fasting to practice physical submission to spiritual goals.
- Recognize that caring for your body is caring for the temple of the Holy Spirit.

The Compounding Effect

Train one arena well, and the others benefit. A strong soul improves emotional regulation, which improves decision-making, which improves physical health. A strong body improves sleep, which improves mental clarity, which improves spiritual focus. The system is interconnected. Optimize one part, and the whole system improves.

You've built practices, structures, and integration. Now you need to measure progress. The next section shows you how to track spiritual growth without becoming legalistic.

PRACTICE PROMPT

- ❖ Identify your weakest arena (heart, mind, body, or soul).
- ❖ For the next month, strengthen that arena while maintaining your spiritual practices.
- ❖ Track how improving one area affects the others.

Here is an example: "My body is my weakest arena. This month, I'll add three strength training sessions per week while maintaining my forty-minute morning spiritual block. I'll track how better sleep and physical energy affect my prayer focus and emotional stability."

Success Criteria

□ You strengthened your weak arena while maintaining your spiritual structure.
□ You noticed and documented specific cross-arena improvements.

Troubleshooting

If you're struggling to maintain both, you're trying to change too much at once. Pick one thing. Do it well. Add the next thing only after the first is automatic.

MEASURING SPIRITUAL PROGRESS

Spiritual growth is real, measurable, and observable. You're not guessing whether you're maturing. You're tracking concrete markers.

Fruit of the Spirit as Scorecard

Galatians 5:22–23 gives you nine measurable categories: love, joy, peace, patience, kindness, goodness, faithfulness, gentleness, self-control.

The Assessment

Rate yourself 1–10 in each category. Be brutally honest. Ask someone who knows you well to rate you as well. Compare the scores they give you with the ones you gave yourself.

If your self-rating is consistently higher than others' ratings, you have a blind spot.

If your ratings are improving quarter over quarter, you're growing.

Discipline Consistency

How often are you doing your spiritual practices? This is the most objective measure for each:

- Scripture reading: Days per week

- Prayer: Minutes per day
- Worship: Attendance percentage
- Fasting: Frequency per month
- Small group: Attendance percentage
- Service: Hours per month

If your metrics are improving or holding steady at a high level, you're on track. If they're declining, something's wrong.

Conviction Speed

How quickly does the Holy Spirit convict you of sin? A healthy soul recognizes sin faster and responds faster.

When you sin, how long does it take you to recognize it, confess it, and repent of it? If the gap is shrinking, your spiritual sensitivity is increasing.

A dull conscience is a dangerous conscience. If you're rationalizing sin or justifying compromise, your soul is weakening.

Service Capacity

Can you serve others without burnout? Spiritual health increases capacity. Spiritual depletion decreases it.

How many hours per week can you serve before you feel resentful, exhausted, or empty? If that number is increasing, your soul is strengthening. If it's decreasing, you're drawing on reserves that aren't being replenished.

Relational Fruit

Are your relationships improving? A strong soul produces a better spouse, better parent, better friend, and better colleague.

Ask the people closest to you, "Am I easier to be around than I was six months ago?" Their answer is data. If they say yes, you're growing. If they hesitate or say no, something needs attention.

Resistance to Temptation

Are you winning battles you used to lose? Spiritual strength shows up in moral victories.

What sin are you struggling with? Are you resisting it more successfully than six months ago? Are you falling less frequently? Recovering faster?

Progress isn't perfection. Progress is trajectory. Are you moving toward holiness or away from it?

You have the framework. You have the practices. You have the measurement tools. Now it's time to commit.

PRACTICE PROMPT

Every three months, do a comprehensive soul audit:

- ❖ Review the fruit of the Spirit. Rate yourself 1–10 on each.

- ❖ Identify your strongest fruit and your weakest fruit.

- ❖ Write one specific practice to strengthen your weakest fruit this quarter.

Here is an example: "Patience is my weakest (rated 4/10). This quarter, I'll pray specifically for patience every morning and practice the ten-second pause before responding when triggered."

- ❖ Rate yourself again in three months.

- ❖ Track the changes.

Success Criteria

☐ You completed the audit honestly and implemented the practice for eighty percent of the quarter.

Troubleshooting

If you see no improvement, examine your practice. Are you doing it consistently? Are you doing it correctly? Are you being specific enough? Vague practice produces vague results.

CONCLUSION

Your soul is the power source for your entire life. Neglect it, and you will collapse. Tend it, and you will thrive.

This is survival. Every person whose life imploded spiritually started the same way: they stopped tending their soul. They got busy. They rationalized and drifted. One day they woke up empty, and they couldn't figure out why.

The blueprint is now in your hands. You have the practices, warnings, and resources. You have the community structures and integration framework.

What you don't have is more time to decide.

Every day you delay is a day of corrosion. Right now, your soul is keeping score, and your body and relationships are feeling the effects. Your capacity to serve is also being determined.

THE FRAMEWORK

Receive. Reflect. Respond. Repeat.

Receive truth through Scripture, prayer, worship, and community. Reflect on truth through meditation, journaling, and contemplation. Respond to truth through obedience, service, repentance, and witness. Repeat the pattern through daily, weekly, and monthly practices.

How Soul Strengthens the Whole SCAL Method

Spiritual disciplines stabilize emotions and build regulation capacity for a sound heart. Spiritual practices require cognitive discipline and sharpen critical thinking for a sound mind. A restored soul improves sleep, immunity, and physical recovery for a strong body. The foundation that everything else flows from is a strong soul.

Your soul is the power source for your entire life. Train it. Tend it. Steward it daily.

The fruit will be life: for you, for your relationships, for your witness, and for the generations that come after you.

Do not delay. Do not rationalize. Start today.

Tomorrow morning, set your alarm forty minutes early. Do all four practices.

Then do it again the next day, and the day after that.

Six months from now, you'll look back and realize that the single best decision you made was to stop treating your soul like an afterthought.

The stakes are eternal. The time is now. Begin.

CHAPTER FIVE
ENDURANCE & STRATEGIC DISCOMFORT

UNDERSTANDING ENDURANCE

My wife's water broke at thirty-three weeks—way too early. We rushed to the hospital, but this was October 2020, and COVID restrictions were in full force. My oldest son, seven years old at the time, wasn't allowed on the maternity floor. I was barely allowed on the floor myself.

We sat in the car, waiting. My wife was contracting in the hospital room. Our baby's life was in danger. And we had to wait forty-five minutes for my parents to drive across town to pick up our oldest before I could even get inside.

When I finally made it in, the nurses prepped us for an emergency C-section. Our son's heart rate kept dropping. Every few minutes, the monitor would alarm. Drop. Recover. Drop. Recover. They moved fast.

I heard his screams when they pulled him out, but they rushed him away before I could see him. The umbilical cord had been wrapped around his neck. Every time my wife contracted, it choked the life out of him. He was also breech. During one hard contraction, he kicked. He literally kicked his way out.

My wife was resting after the procedure when the nurses noticed something. The left side of her face had gone slack.

They tried not to sound alarmed, but I could see it in their eyes. They rushed her down to the ICU (intensive care unit). Stroke was suspected.

So there I was, running all over the hospital. The ICU to check on my wife. The neonatal intensive care unit (NICU) to check on my son. Back and forth. I saw my little guy in the NICU—so fragile, so small, tubes running into his tiny body. I saw my wife in the ICU—exhausted, worried, her face not looking the same.

Eventually, the doctors cleared her. It was not a stroke. The diagnosis was Bells Palsy, thought to have been from severe exhaustion and stress. Our son stayed in the NICU.

The day we left the hospital without him was the hardest moment of my life, or so I thought. The next five weeks would prove much harder.

My wife and oldest son were home. I had to go back to work at my 9–5 job. I was also running the studio. Times were rough. My schedule looked like this:

5:00 AM: Wake up and work remotely.
9:00 AM–5:00 PM: Do the day job.
5:30 PM–8:30 PM: Go to the studio and train clients.
9:00 PM–12:00 AM: Sit at the hospital with my son, passing on love from me, his mom, and his brother.
12:30 AM: Drive home.
1:00 AM: Shower.
1:30 AM: Go to bed.
5:00 AM: Repeat.

I lived like that for five weeks. Around week two, instinctually, I pressed the big red button that read "auto-pilot." It was the only way I could be where I needed to be for everyone who needed me.

I had to put up walls.

I stopped myself from feeling. I couldn't *afford* to feel. Feeling the weight of what was happening would have caused me to break down. That couldn't happen. My wife needed me strong. My oldest needed me present, and my son in the NICU needed me to show up every night. The studio needed me functional, and my job needed me performing.

So I became a robot.

I didn't pray—not really. I didn't talk about how it felt. Rather than process anything, I just kept moving, executing the schedule. Hospital. Studio. Work. Home. Repeat. I smiled at clients and answered emails. I sat with my son in the NICU and talked to him like everything was fine. Then I came home and played with my oldest like I wasn't running on three hours of sleep.

Everyone needed me. I couldn't falter, not a single bit.

And I didn't.

I made it through all five weeks. My son came home. Thank God he didn't have many challenges ahead. He was growing. Safe.

I thought I'd feel relief. I did, But I also felt . . . nothing.

The problem with shutting everything down is that I didn't even know I'd done it until well after my son was home safe. I shut it all down to survive and never turned it back on.

I didn't know the word *hupomone* then. I didn't know that what I was doing had a name in Scripture: remaining under the load. I just knew quitting wasn't an option, so I survived the only way I knew how: by shutting off everything that would slow me down. Feelings. Connection. Presence. I became a machine because machines don't break. At least, that's what I thought. Cut me some slack here. I was running on three hours of sleep a night. Thinking around that time wasn't my strong suit.

But here's what I didn't know then: you can't stay a machine. Eventually, you have to feel again. And when you do, everything you avoided comes crashing down at once.

This chapter is about building endurance so when the next trial comes—and it will—you don't have to shut down to survive. You remain human while remaining under the load. That's what I didn't know how to do. That's what I'm going to teach you.

Endurance and stamina are different. Typically, the way I coach it is this: stamina is what you have before you hit adverse conditions. It's the measure of your energy output before you're tired. Endurance is what happens after you're tired, how much further you can go when everything in you wants to quit.

This distinction matters. Stamina gets you to the hard part. Endurance gets you through it.

Endurance is the ability to continue or last despite fatigue, stress, or other adverse conditions. It is the ability to bear pain and hardships.

Here's what most people miss: you cannot build endurance without strategic discomfort. You cannot strengthen what you never test. The body, the mind, the heart, and the soul all require resistance to grow. Without it, they atrophy.

"And not only so, but we glory in tribulations also, knowing that tribulation worketh patience; and patience, experience; and experience, hope" (Romans 5:3–4).

This verse tells us that tribulation produces endurance. Experience builds on that endurance. Hope emerges from proven character forged through testing.

This is the pattern: adversity, adaptation, advancement. The Christian life is not about comfort. It's about becoming capable of carrying what God calls you to carry.

Hebrews 12:1 presses the point further.

"Wherefore seeing we also are compassed about with so great a cloud of witnesses, let us lay aside every weight, and the sin which doth so easily beset us, and let us run with patience the race that is set before us."(Hebrews 12:1).

Run with patience. That's endurance language. The race is long. The weight is real, and the sin is persistent. The only way through is to train yourself to last.

THE GREEK: HUPOMONE

The Greek word translated as "endurance" or "patience" in Romans 5:3–4 is *hupomone* (ὑπομονή). The word is composed of two parts: *hupo* meaning "under" and *meno* meaning "to abide, remain." Literally: "to remain under."

This is not passive waiting. This is active perseverance under load. It's the capacity to bear weight without collapse and stay in position when everything in you screams, "Run."

Hupomone appears thirty-two times in the New Testament, and it is always in contexts of sustained pressure: trials, persecution, tribulation, and affliction. It describes the person who carries the burden faithfully, one who doesn't throw off the load when it gets heavy.

This is different from *makrothumia* (patience toward people) or *karteria* (patient endurance in suffering). *Hupomone* is specifically about remaining under the load. It is not removing the load, numbing yourself to it, or pretending it isn't there; it means carrying it faithfully until the work is done.

HOW THIS CONNECTS

You've spent four chapters building your foundation.
The Heart chapter taught you to regulate emotions:
Name → Accept → Analyze → Express → Reframe.
The Mind chapter showed you how to think clearly:
Perceive → Comprehend → Evaluate → Decide → Act.
The Body chapter gave you tools for your physicality:
Train → Recover → Adapt → Repeat.
The Soul chapter established the path to spiritual health:
Receive → Reflect → Respond → Repeat.

Each framework works. Each one builds capacity. But here's what you need to understand: they collapse under sustained pressure unless you've built endurance across all four arenas.

Emotional regulation works until you're exhausted, then your Heart framework fails. Mental clarity holds until decision fatigue sets in, then your Mind framework fails. Physical discipline sustains until recovery can't keep pace, then your Body framework fails. Spiritual practices continue until God feels distant for months, then your Soul framework fails.

Endurance is what keeps the frameworks functional when conditions turn hostile. It trains you to tolerate intense emotions without being ruled by them. You can feel anger without acting in rage, grieve without collapsing. It builds your capacity to think clearly under pressure. When circumstances are chaotic, you stay sharp; when fatigue sets in, you keep reasoning. It conditions your body to perform when depleted: recovery improves, resilience deepens, you become harder to break. It develops your ability to work through pain, hardships, and trials while leaning on God for strength, without wavering in your faith and without compromising on what is true.

What unites all of these? Strategic discomfort. Deliberately choose to get uncomfortable on purpose, so that when real adversity comes, you're already conditioned to endure.

The question isn't whether you'll face trials. The question is whether you'll have built the capacity to endure them.

THE CALL TO ENDURE

Scripture does not romanticize suffering. It commands endurance through it. James 1:2–3 sets the tone:

"My brethren, count it all joy when ye fall into divers temptations; knowing this, that the trying of your faith worketh patience" (James 1:2–3).

The testing of faith produces endurance. It does not produce comfort or ease. Trials reveal what you're made of and forge what you're becoming. James 4:7 follows with instruction for this:

"Submit yourselves therefore to God. Resist the devil, and he will flee from you"(James 4:7).

Resistance requires endurance. You don't resist evil once and call it done. You resist it repeatedly, consistently, until the pattern of obedience becomes second nature. Romans 12:12 adds clarity:

"Rejoicing in hope; patient in tribulation; continuing instant in prayer"(Romans 12:12).

Be patient in tribulation. Don't be numb or passive. Have patience. Stay steady when everything around you is falling apart. That's spiritual endurance.

The Romans 5 Progression

Romans 5:3–5 gives us the complete sequence:

"And not only so, but we glory in tribulations also: knowing that tribulation worketh patience; And patience, experience;

and experience, hope: And hope maketh not ashamed; because the love of God is shed abroad in our hearts by the Holy Ghost which is given unto us" (Romans 5:3–5).

Let's break this down word by word, because every part matters.

Thlipsis (tribulation): Pressure, affliction, distress. External forces squeeze you. This is not about minor inconveniences but real hardship that tests everything.

Hupomone (patience/endurance): That word again. Remaining under the load. Sustaining effort despite opposition. Tribulation produces this if you don't quit.

Dokime (experience): Proven character. The Greek carries the sense of something tested and approved, like metal refined by fire. This is the character that remains after the impurities are burned away—not theoretical virtue, but character demonstrated under pressure.

Elpis (hope): Not wishful thinking, Biblical hope is confident expectation rooted in God's faithfulness. It's the assurance that God is working all things for your good, even when you can't see it yet.

Paul isn't giving you a motivational speech. He's describing a spiritual law: pressure produces perseverance; perseverance produces proven character; proven character produces confident hope.

You can't skip steps. You can't manufacture hope without going through the fire first.

The Wilderness Training Ground

Scripture reveals God's method:

"And thou shalt remember all the way which the LORD thy God led thee these forty years in the wilderness, to humble thee, and to prove thee, to know what was in thine heart, whether thou wouldest keep his commandments, or no" (Deuteronomy 8:2).

The wilderness wasn't punishment. It was a training ground.

God led Israel through forty years of hardship to reveal what was in their hearts and to build the endurance they would need for the Promised Land. The journey from Egypt to Canaan should have taken eleven days (Deuteronomy 1:2). It took forty years because they weren't ready. They had the stamina to leave Egypt, but they lacked the endurance needed to enter Canaan.

The wilderness built what Egypt couldn't: a generation capable of enduring what conquest would require.

God does the same with you.

The trials you face aren't random. They're designed to build endurance you'll need for what's ahead. The question is this: will you endure the training, or will you quit in the wilderness?

This is the biblical foundation for strategic discomfort. God uses trials to build endurance. You can cooperate with that process by voluntarily choosing difficulty, or you can resist it and stay weak. Either way, the trials will come. The only question is whether you'll be ready.

THE SHIFT TO FRAGILITY

Alicia's grandfather could work 12-hour days in a factory, come home and work on the farm, and still have energy for his family. At age forty-two, her grandfather was stronger than Alicia is now.

What changed?

Modern life removed most physical, mental, and emotional demands that used to build endurance automatically. Comfort became the default. And comfort, unchecked, creates fragility.

Consider what's been removed from most people's daily life, in just two generations:

Physical labor used to be unavoidable. People walked miles to work, lifted heavy things daily, and worked with their hands. Bodies adapted because survival required it. Now? Alicia drives everywhere, sits at a desk, and orders food to her door. Her body has no reason to stay strong.

Mental challenge used to be constant. One had to navigate without GPS, do math without calculators, remember phone numbers and addresses, and solve problems without Google. Brains stayed sharp because daily life demanded it. Now? Alicia outsources most cognitive work to her phone. Her brain has atrophied from disuse.

Emotional resilience used to be built through unavoidable hardship. Death was closer. Loss was common. Conflict couldn't be avoided. People learned to sit with grief, navigate tension, and process pain because there was no other option. Now? Alicia can numb any uncomfortable emotion within seconds. Scroll, binge, shop, eat. Discomfort is optional.

Spiritual discipline used to be reinforced by community and necessity. Church wasn't a choice; it was how a person stayed connected to their community. Scripture reading and prayer were habits passed down and expected. Now? Alicia's spiritual life is entirely self-motivated, and when motivation fades, so does her practice.

The result is that Alicia has inherited none of the endurance her grandfather built. The demands were unavoidable, so adaptation was automatic. Alicia has low tolerance because life doesn't demand it and she hasn't voluntarily chosen to raise the bar. Modern comfort has removed the automatic adaptation triggers, leaving her weak.

Example: Alicia's Fragility

Alicia is a project manager at a mid-sized firm. She has been married to Marcus for fifteen years. She is the mother of three kids: ages twelve, nine, and six. She goes to church most Sundays. She wants to be a good wife, a present mother, and a faithful servant of God.

But Alicia is tired. All the time.

She's not athletic, and never has been. She can start things—new workout programs, new diets, new spiritual disciplines—but she can't sustain them. When things get hard, she quits. When workouts get uncomfortable, she stops. When conversations get tense, she withdraws. When prayer feels dry, she skips it. When projects at work get complicated, she procrastinates.

Alicia's problem isn't that she's weak. Her problem is that she quits too soon.

She has stamina. She can start strong. But she lacks endurance, the capacity to continue when the load gets heavy. That lack shows up everywhere.

Her body is declining. At forty-two, she's winded walking up two flights of stairs. Her back hurts constantly. She's thirty pounds overweight and prediabetic. The doctor's warnings aren't hypothetical anymore; they're urgent. But every time she tries to change, she quits within three weeks.

Her emotions are brittle. A criticism at work from her supervisor doesn't just sting; it ruins her entire day. She replays the conversation for hours, sometimes days. A tense conversation with Marcus leaves her withdrawn and silent for the rest of the evening. She snaps at her kids over small things, then feels crushing guilt afterward.

Her mind gives up under pressure. Complex projects at work overwhelm her. She can focus for maybe firty-five minutes before her attention scatters into email, Slack, her phone. Decision fatigue hits hard by midafternoon. By evening, she's mentally exhausted and can barely help her kids with homework.

Her spiritual life is shallow. She prays when she feels like it, which isn't often. Bible reading happens sporadically—she'll go strong for a week after a convicting sermon, then do nothing for two months. When God feels distant, Alicia drifts. She knows she should be different. She wants to be different. But she doesn't know how.

Alicia represents most of us: people who want to serve well but are running on fumes, who start strong but fade fast, who lack the endurance to finish what they start.

The Fragility Cascade

Low endurance in one arena weakens the others. This isn't theoretical; it's physiological and psychological reality.

Physical fragility leads to mental decline. Sedentary lifestyle reduces BDNF, weakening memory and learning. Poor cardiovascular fitness reduces oxygen delivery to the brain, slowing processing speed. Lack of physical challenge reduces stress resilience, making mental work feel harder.

Mental fragility creates emotional brittleness. Weak executive function (from lack of mental training) reduces impulse control. Poor focus habits make it harder to sit with uncomfortable emotions. Mental fatigue from shallow thinking reduces capacity for emotional regulation.

Emotional brittleness produces spiritual shallowness. Inability to tolerate difficult emotions leads to avoiding hard spiritual truths. Emotional reactivity prevents the stillness required for prayer and reflection. Fear of discomfort leads to avoiding spiritual disciplines: fasting, confession, confrontation. Spiritual shallowness results in physical neglect. Lack of transcendent purpose removes motivation for physical discipline. Shallow faith produces short-term thinking, neglecting long-term stewardship. Spiritual drift removes the conviction that the body is a temple requiring care.

The cascade accelerates. Fragility breeds more fragility. Weakness in one arena makes you weaker everywhere.

Alicia's life demonstrates this. She stopped working out (physical fragility). Her mind became foggier (mental decline). Her emotions became more reactive (emotional brittleness). Her prayer life dried up (spiritual shallowness). Now every arena is weak, and each weakness reinforces the others.

STRATEGIC DISCOMFORT

If comfort creates fragility, then strategic discomfort creates resilience. Strategic discomfort is controlled exposure to difficulty across all four arenas, designed to build endurance capacity that transfers everywhere.

Just as exposure to a controlled dose of a pathogen can build immunity, strategic discomfort exposes you to controlled doses of hardship to build resilience.

Choose the hard thing. Control the dose. Do it consistently, and over time, your capacity grows.

CAPACITY THAT TRANSFERS

The Body chapter gave you the complete framework: Train → Recover → Adapt → Repeat.

You learned resistance training protocols, weekly templates, and recovery modalities. Now we're building on that foundation with endurance-specific training and how physical capacity transfers to mental, emotional, and spiritual strength.

You're not relearning the body. You're learning how to build the specific type of physical capacity that makes you harder to break everywhere.

Example: Alicia's Physical Baseline

Alicia can lift weights for a forty-five-minute session. She has decent strength for an untrained forty-two-year-old person. But ask her to run for twenty minutes, and it's different. She's gasping, heart rate spiking to 180 beats per minute. By minute eight, she's ready to quit.

Strength asks, "How much can you lift once?"

Endurance asks, "How long can you keep going?"

Alicia has some strength. She has almost no endurance.

The Endurance Adaptation

When you train for endurance, your body makes specific adaptations that are distinct from strength training:

- **Mitochondrial Biogenesis is the process by which** your cells create more mitochondria (the energy factories of the cell). More mitochondria means more sustained energy production.
- **Increased Capillary Density** means more blood vessels form around muscle fibers, improving oxygen and nutrient delivery.
- **Enhanced Lactate Buffering** makes your body get better at clearing and tolerating the acidic buildup that causes that burning sensation in muscles.
- **Improved Fat Utilization** leads to your body becoming more efficient at using fat for fuel instead of relying solely on glycogen (stored carbs).
- **Stroke Volume Increase** makes your heart more efficient; it pumps more blood per beat, which lowers resting heart rate and improves cardiovascular efficiency.

This is the translation: Endurance training makes you harder to exhaust. Your energy systems become more efficient. Your cardiovascular system becomes stronger. You can sustain effort longer before fatigue sets in.

Alicia's Physical Endurance Protocol

Alicia starts with baseline cardiovascular work. It's nothing fancy. Just consistent, progressive exposure.

Weeks One Through Four: Building the Base

- **Frequency:** Three times per week, a twenty-minute session (run, bike, row, or brisk walk)
- **Target:** Conversational pace (able to speak in full sentences)
- **Heart rate:** Sixty to seventy percent of max (roughly 130–145 bpm for Alicia)
- **Goal:** Being able to finish each session without walking

Week one is brutal. Alicia completes twenty minutes, but barely. She wants to quit at minute twelve. Her heart rate spikes to 165 beats per minute. She walks twice, but she finishes. The first night, she writes in her journal: "Pathetic. I used to be able to do this." The shame burns, but she commits to showing up again.

Week two still feels hard. The quit urge hits at minute fourteen. Heart rate stays around 155. She only walks once. She notices something: the urge to quit feels the same, but she's lasting two minutes longer before it hits.

Week three brings a shift. Quit urge hits at minute sixteen. Heart rate is 150. No walking breaks. Alicia starts to believe maybe she can actually do this.

By week four, the quit urge doesn't hit until minute eighteen. She finishes strong. Heart rate is 145. For the first time in months, she feels capable. Not strong yet but capable.

Here's her progress: The quit point moved from minute twelve to minute eighteen. That's endurance-building.

Weeks Five Through Eight: Increasing Duration

- Same frequency but with thirty-minute sessions
- Same conversational pace
- Same target heart rate of sixty to seventy percent of max

Week five: Thirty minutes feels brutal. Quit urge hit at minute twenty. But Alicia pushes through. She remembers what her pastor said in a sermon two months prior: "The point where you want to quit is the point where growth begins." She didn't understand it then. She understands it now.

Week eight: Thirty minutes feels manageable. The quit urge doesn't hit until minute twenty-seven. Heart rate stays stable at 140. Alicia notices she's not as winded going up the stairs at work. Her kids notice she's less irritable in the evenings.

Weeks Nine Through Twelve: Adding Intensity

- Twice per week: 30-minute steady-state (conversational pace)
- Once per week: 20-minute interval session (1 minute hard, 2 minutes easy, repeat)

The interval work teaches the body to recover quickly and tolerate higher intensity. Alicia's heart rate spikes to 175 during hard intervals but drops to 130 during recovery. Her body learns to buffer lactate and clear metabolic waste faster.

Week Twelve Result

Alicia can now run thirty-five minutes at a conversational pace without wanting to quit. Her resting heart rate dropped from seventy-eight to sixty-eight beats per minute. Her recovery time after hard sessions went from seventy-two hours to thirty-six hours. She's not an endurance athlete, but she's no longer fragile.

More importantly, Alicia notices something unexpected. Her mental endurance improved. Her emotional resilience increased. Her spiritual disciplines became easier to maintain. Physical endurance transferred to other life arenas.

The Transfer Mechanism

Physical endurance builds more than cardiovascular fitness; it builds psychological resilience.

Every time Alicia pushed through the quit urge during a run, she practiced tolerating discomfort. That skill transferred. When work stress hit, she didn't collapse as quickly. When conversations with Marcus got tense, she could sit in the discomfort longer. When prayer felt dry, she kept going instead of quitting.

The mechanism is **self-efficacy.** Each time you do a hard

thing, you prove to yourself that you can. That proof transfers to other domains. You start believing, "If I can endure this, I can endure that."

Research confirms this. Studies on grit and perseverance show that endurance built in one domain increases perseverance in unrelated domains. The brain doesn't compartmentalize endurance. It generalizes it.

Train physical endurance, and you build a bias toward persistence everywhere.

PRACTICE PROMPT

❖ Choose one endurance-building session this week: 20-minute run, 30-minute bike, 45-minute hike, or 20-minute rowing.

❖ Track three things:
  - When the quit urge hits (at which minute/mile?)
  - How you talk yourself through it
  - How you feel thirty minutes post-session

❖ Repeat weekly for 4 weeks. Track how the quit point moves.

Success Criteria

☐ You completed one endurance session this week and tracked when the quit urge hit.
☐ You wrote down how you talked yourself through it.
☐ You noted how you felt thirty minutes after.
☐ You committed to repeating this weekly for four weeks while tracking the quit point's movement.

Troubleshooting

If you couldn't identify when the quit urge hit, it either came so early you didn't notice, or you didn't push hard enough. Next time, pay closer attention to the moment you first think, *I want to stop.*

If you didn't talk yourself through anything, you either stopped immediately or pushed through on autopilot. Practice one simple phrase: "Just five more minutes."

If you felt terrible thirty minutes post-session, you either went too hard (scale back intensity) or didn't hydrate/fuel properly.

If the quit point hasn't moved after four weeks, you're not being consistent enough. Did you actually do it weekly?

BUILDING COGNITIVE STAMINA

The Mind chapter taught you Perceive → Comprehend → Evaluate → Decide → Act. You learned critical thinking strategies, how to cut toxicity, and how to spot fallacies. Now we're building sustained cognitive capacity: the ability to think clearly under fatigue and pressure.

Intelligence is your processing power. Mental endurance is how long you can sustain that processing power before exhaustion degrades performance.

Example: Alicia's Mental Baseline

Alicia can focus deeply for about forty-five minutes. After that, her attention starts to scatter. Complex problems feel overwhelming. Decision fatigue hits hard around mid-afternoon.

This is normal for most people. But normal doesn't mean optimal.

Alicia isn't dumb. She's mentally weak. Her mind gives up too soon.

The Mental Fatigue Problem

Mental work depletes cognitive resources. Specifically, it depletes glucose and neurotransmitters in the prefrontal cortex (the part of the brain responsible for focus, planning, and decision-making).

When the prefrontal cortex fatigues, these things tend to happen:

- Focus deteriorates.
- Decision quality declines.
- Impulse control weakens.
- Complex reasoning becomes difficult.

You make worse decisions at the end of the day than at the beginning because your prefrontal cortex is depleted.

Building mental endurance means the prefrontal cortex can sustain effort longer before fatigue sets in.

Alicia's Mental Endurance Protocol

Alicia's approach: Progressive exposure to sustained cognitive work.

Weeks One Through Four: Building Focus Stamina

- Five days per week: sixty-minute deep work session (one complex task, no distractions)
- Rule: No phone, no email, no interruptions
- Track: When the quit urge hits

Week one: Quit urge at thirty-five minutes. Alicia pushes to forty-five minutes. Barely. She feels her brain screaming for distraction. Her hand reaches for her phone three times. She catches herself each time.

Week two: Quit urge at forty minutes. Pushes to fifty minutes. The resistance is still intense, but she's learning to recognize it without obeying it.

Week three: Quit urge at forty-five minutes. Pushes to sixty minutes. For the first time, she completes the full hour. The last fifteen minutes are torture, but she does it.

Week four: Quit urge at fifty-five minutes. Completes sixty minutes feeling strong. She notices the quality of her work is higher when she sustains focus this long.

Progress: The quit point moved from thirty-five to fifty-five minutes. Mental endurance is building.

Weeks Five Through Eight: Increasing Duration and Complexity

- Five days per week: ninety-minute deep work session
- Rule: Same (no distractions)
- Added challenge: Tackle more complex problems during these sessions.

Week five: Ninety minutes feels brutal. Quit urge at sixty

minutes. But Alicia finishes. Her brain feels fried afterward, but she did it.

Week eight: Ninety minutes feels manageable. Quit urge doesn't hit until minute seventy-five. Alicia is solving problems in this deep state that she couldn't touch when her focus was fragmented.

Weeks Nine Through Twelve: Adding Cognitive Load Under Fatigue

- Three days per week: two-hour deep work session
- Two days per week: ninety-minute session + thirty-minute problem-solving under fatigue (intentionally tackling hard problems when tired)

The fatigue training matters. Most of life requires you to think clearly when you're already tired. Training cognitive function under fatigue builds resilience that transfers to real-world pressure.

Week 12 Result

Alicia can now sustain deep focus for two hours without significant degradation. Complex problem-solving under fatigue improved dramatically. Decision quality late in the day increased. She's not a genius, but her mind no longer quits on her.

And again, the transfer effect shows up. Alicia noticed that her emotional regulation improved. When her kids acted up late in the evening, she didn't snap as quickly. Her patience extended. Her prefrontal cortex was stronger, so impulse control improved across the board.

The Science: Executive Function and Endurance

Executive function (the brain's ability to plan, focus, and regulate behavior) is trainable. Like a muscle, it strengthens with use.

Research on cognitive training shows the following:

- Sustained attention improves with practice.
- Working memory capacity increases with training.
- Cognitive control (the ability to override impulses) strengthens through repeated use.

Your brain adapts to the demands you place on it. If you only ask it to focus for twenty minutes, it will remain weak. If you consistently push it to ninety minutes, two hours, or longer, it adapts.

Mental endurance is not fixed, and training it has cascading effects on every other arena.

PRACTICE PROMPT

Choose one mentally demanding task that typically makes you quit around the two-hour mark. This week, when you hit that quit point, take a five-minute break (walk, breathe, water), then come back for thirty more minutes.

Track these:

- When the quit urge hit
- What you did during the break
- How the final thirty minutes felt
- Whether you finished the task

Repeat weekly. Notice how the quit point gradually moves later.

Success Criteria

☐ You identified one mentally demanding task.
☐ You worked until you hit your quit point, took a five-minute break, and returned for thirty more minutes.
☐ You tracked all four elements.☐ You committed to repeating this weekly.

Troubleshooting

If the quit urge never hit, you're not working on something truly demanding. Pick a harder task.

If you took the break but couldn't return, thirty minutes was too ambitious. Try ten minutes first.

If the final thirty minutes felt impossible, your break wasn't restorative enough. Try walking outside or doing light stretching.

If you finished the task before the thirty minutes were up, excellent. That's progress. Next week, push fifteen minutes past your quit point instead of taking a break.

EMOTIONAL ENDURANCE

The Heart chapter taught you Name → Accept → Analyze → Express → Reframe. You learned how to regulate emotions, identify triggers, and process difficult feelings. Now we're building the capacity to sit with intense emotions for extended periods without numbing, avoiding, or being ruled by them.

Emotional intelligence gives you the tools. Emotional endurance gives you the stamina to use those tools when emotions run hot.

Example: Alicia's Emotional Baseline

Alicia avoids emotional discomfort at all costs.

A critical email from her boss doesn't just bother her; it devastates her. She can't let it go. She rereads it fifteen times, crafting responses she'll never send. The rest of her workday is shot. A tense conversation with Marcus about their finances leaves her withdrawn and silent for hours, sometimes the whole next day. When her kids push back on discipline, she either snaps in anger or withdraws in frustration. There's no middle ground.

Her problem isn't that she feels emotions. She can't tolerate them. The moment discomfort hits, she either explodes or numbs. She scrolls her phone. She eats. She avoids. She does anything except sit with what she's feeling.

Emotional endurance is the capacity to stay present with difficult emotions without being controlled by them or shutting them down. It is to feel anger without acting in rage, to grieve without collapsing, to experience anxiety without panicking.

Alicia has none of this. Her emotional tolerance is near zero.

The Emotional Avoidance Problem

When you avoid difficult emotions, you never build the capacity to tolerate them. And avoidance is easier than ever.

Feel bored? Scroll your phone. Feel anxious? Binge a show. Feel grief? Eat, shop, work, distract. Within seconds, you can numb any uncomfortable emotion.

But here's the problem: avoidance doesn't eliminate the emotion. It just delays it. And every time you avoid, you reinforce the belief that the emotion is intolerable.

Over time, your emotional tolerance shrinks. What used to be manageable now feels overwhelming. You become emotionally fragile.

This is Alicia's avoidance pattern:

- Alicia receives criticism at work, withdraws, and avoids the person for days.
- There is tension with Marcus, and Alicia goes silent, scrolls on her phone, and avoids conversation.
- When she experiences frustration with her kids, she yells or walks away.

Alicia never practices sitting with discomfort, so her capacity never grows.

Alicia's Emotional Endurance Protocol

Alicia's approach is to deliberately practice sitting with uncomfortable emotions instead of avoiding them.

Weeks One Through Four: Naming and Sitting

- **Daily practice:** When an uncomfortable emotion hits, name it and sit with it for five minutes before taking any action.
- **Rule:** No phone, no distraction, no numbing is allowed.
- **Track** which emotion, the intensity (1–10), and how long until the urge to avoid hit.

Week one, she feels anxiety about a work presentation. Intensity: 7/10. Urge to scroll hits at two minutes. Alicia forces herself to sit for five minutes. It's excruciating. Her chest tightens. Her breathing gets shallow. She wants to run. But she stays. When the timer goes off, the intensity has dropped to 5/10. She's shaking, but she did it.

Week two, frustration with her nine-year-old daughter's attitude mounts. Intensity: 6/10. The urge to yell hits immediately. Alicia names it out loud: "I'm feeling frustrated and disrespected." She sits with it for five minutes. The intensity drops to 4/10. When she finally responds, her voice is calm, not sharp.

Week three, grief about her father's declining health hits. Intensity: 8/10. The urge to distract hits at one minute. Alicia sits with it. She cries for three minutes straight—deep, wrenching sobs. Then the emotion passes. Not gone, but manageable.

Week four, Marcus criticizes how she handled a parenting situation. Intensity: 7/10. The urge to defend herself hits immediately. Alicia names it: "I'm feeling defensive and hurt." She sits with it for five minutes. Then she responds calmly: "You're right. I could have handled that better."

Progress: Alicia's emotional tolerance is increasing. Emotions that used to feel unbearable now feel difficult but manageable.

Weeks Five Through Eight: Extending the Sit Time

- Daily practice: Sit with uncomfortable emotions for 10 minutes before responding.
- Added challenge: Practice this during high-intensity situations (not just mild discomfort).

Week five, there is a major work conflict with a colleague who undermined her in a meeting. Intensity: 9/10. Sit time: ten minutes. Alicia writes out what she's feeling instead of immediately responding. Her written response is measured, not reactive. She sends the email the next day, not in the heat of anger.

Week eight, a tense conversation with Marcus about finances takes place. Intensity: 8/10. Alicia sits with the defensiveness and anxiety for ten minutes. Then she engages in the conversation without shutting down or attacking. The conversation is hard but productive. They actually resolve something instead of just fighting.

Weeks Nine Through Twelve: Practicing Emotional Endurance Under Compounding Stress

- Daily practice: Same (ten-minute sit time)
- Added challenge: Intentionally have difficult conversations at the end of long days (when emotional regulation is hardest).

Week twelve, Alicia's emotional tolerance has increased dramatically. Emotions that used to trigger immediate avoidance or explosion now trigger curiosity. She can sit with anger, anxiety, grief, and frustration without being ruled by them.

And here's the transfer effect: Her relationships improved.

Marcus noticed she wasn't withdrawing as much. Her kids noticed she wasn't snapping as often. Her coworkers noticed she wasn't as reactive to feedback. One colleague even asked, "What's different about you lately? You seem calmer."

Emotional endurance didn't eliminate difficult emotions. It built the capacity to remain present with them.

DISTRESS TOLERANCE

Research on Dialectical Behavior Therapy (DBT) shows that distress tolerance is a trainable skill. The more you practice sitting with discomfort, the stronger your capacity becomes.

Brain imaging studies reveal that naming emotions ("affect labeling") reduces activation of the amygdala (the brain's fear center) and increases activity in the prefrontal cortex (the brain's rational center). Translation: When you name what you're feeling and sit with it, you literally calm your nervous system.

Emotional endurance matters because it builds the neurological capacity to stay regulated when emotions run high.

As with physical and mental endurance, emotional endurance transfers. Train it in low-stakes situations, and you'll have it available in high-stakes moments.

PRACTICE PROMPT

Anytime you feel intense emotion (7/10 or higher), use the protocol:

- ❖ Name the intensity out loud. "I'm feeling [emotion] at a [number] out of ten."

- ❖ Anchor physically. Put your feet on floor and take three deep breaths.

- ❖ Remind yourself, "This won't last forever. I can stay."

- ❖ Stay for five minutes without numbing, distracting, or escaping.

- ❖ Write afterward: What happened? Did the intensity decrease? Did you survive?

❖ Track five instances over the next month. Notice if your tolerance increases.

Success Criteria

☐ You practiced the full protocol during one intense emotion (7/10).
☐ You completed all five steps including the five-minute stay and written reflection.
☐ You tracked five total instances over a month.

Troubleshooting

If you didn't encounter a 7/10+ emotion, either you're emotionally stable (rare) or you're not noticing intensity levels. Try tracking all emotions for a week to calibrate your scale.

If you couldn't name the intensity, practice the skill with lower-intensity emotions first (4/10, 5/10).

If you couldn't stay for five minutes, start with two minutes. The goal is progress, not perfection.

If the intensity didn't decrease, that's actually fine—the point is learning you can survive it.

If you only tracked one or two instances instead of five, extend your timeline to sixty days.

SPIRITUAL ENDURANCE

The Soul chapter taught you Receive → Reflect → Respond → Repeat. You learned the four foundational practices (Scripture, prayer, worship, fasting), how to build structure, and how to navigate spiritual dryness.

Now we're building the capacity to remain faithful when God feels distant, when obedience costs you something, and when spiritual disciplines feel mechanical.

Spiritual knowledge gives you the framework. Spiritual endurance gives you the capacity to remain faithful when feelings fail you.

Example: Alicia's Spiritual Baseline

Alicia prays when she feels like it, which isn't often. Bible reading happens sporadically. When worship feels alive, she's engaged. When it feels dead, she drifts.

Her spiritual life is entirely feeling-dependent. When God feels close, Alicia is faithful. When God feels distant, Alicia disappears.

Spiritual endurance is the ability to remain faithful to God regardless of how you feel. It lets you do all of these:

- Pray when prayer feels dry.
- Read Scripture when it feels lifeless.
- Worship when you don't feel like it.
- Obey when obedience costs you something.

James 1:12 defines it for us.

"Blessed is the man that endureth temptation: for when he is tried, he shall receive the crown of life, which the Lord hath promised to them that love him" (James 1:12).

We need endurance through temptation and faithfulness through testing. We must continue even when things get hard.

Alicia has none of this. Her faith is a fair-weather faith. And fair-weather faith cannot endure the storms.

The Spiritual Drift Problem

When spiritual disciplines are feeling-dependent, they collapse the moment feelings fade. Feelings always fade.

Prayer will feel dry. Scripture will feel lifeless. Worship will feel dead. Obedience will feel costly. If your faithfulness depends on feeling good, you won't last.

This is Alicia's pattern:

- When she feels spiritually alive after a powerful sermon, she prays daily for a week. Feelings fade. Prayer stops.
- After reading a challenging passage, she feels convicted and commits to daily Bible reading. Discipline feels hard. She stops after ten days.
- Alivia feels close to God during a worship service and engages fully. Next Sunday feels flat, and she stops engaging.

She never builds endurance because she quits the moment discomfort hits.

Alicia's Spiritual Endurance Protocol

Alicia's approach needs to be to commit to spiritual disciplines regardless of how they feel, and to track faithfulness, not feelings.

Weeks One Through Four: Daily Nonnegotiables

- Five minutes of prayer every morning (no exceptions)
- Ten minutes of Scripture reading every evening (no exceptions)
- Rule: Faithfulness to the discipline matters more than how it feels.

Week one, prayer feels forced. Alicia sits in silence for most of the five minutes, unsure what to say. Scripture reading feels dry. The words blur together. But she does it anyway, seven days straight. She writes in her journal: "This feels pointless. Am I doing this wrong?"

Week two, it still feels forced. Alicia wants to quit. "What's the point if I don't feel anything?" But she continues for seven more days. One morning, a phrase from her Scripture reading the night before surfaces while she's making breakfast. It's a small thing, but it surprises her.

Week three, there is a shift. Prayer still feels difficult but less forced. She starts talking to God like He's actually listening. Scripture reading starts connecting. Not every day, but some days. She notices patterns she missed before. Themes emerging across different passages.

Week four, prayer feels conversational on three out of seven days. Scripture reading engages her on four out of seven days. But she keeps the discipline on all seven days, regardless of how it feels. The consistency itself becomes meaningful.

Alicia is building the habit of faithfulness independent of feelings.

Weeks Five Through Eight: Extending the Time

- Ten minutes of prayer every morning
- Fifteen minutes of Scripture reading every evening

- Added challenge: One day per week, fast from lunch (a practice in saying "no" to physical hunger to strengthen spiritual hunger)

Week five, fasting is brutal. Alicia's stomach growls at noon. She's irritable. She snaps at a coworker over email. But she prays during lunch instead of eating. The discomfort sharpens her focus on God in a way that surprises her. She realizes how much she uses food to numb herself.

Week eight, fasting still isn't easy, but it's no longer unbearable. Prayer time occasionally extends past ten minutes because Alicia doesn't want to stop. She's actually talking to God now, not just reciting requests. Scripture reading captivates her five out of seven days. She's underlining passages, writing notes in the margins.

Weeks Nine Through Twelve: Adding Spiritual Disciplines Under Pressure

- Daily prayer and Scripture continue.
- Weekly fasting continues.
- **Added challenge:** Pray at the end of long days when she's exhausted (not just first thing in the morning).

Week 12 Result

Alicia's spiritual life is no longer feeling-dependent. She prays when prayer feels dry. She reads Scripture when it feels lifeless. She worships when she doesn't feel like it. And paradoxically, the more faithful she is regardless of feelings, the more often the feelings return.

More importantly: Alicia's endurance in the other arenas strengthened her spiritual life. Physical endurance taught her to push through discomfort. Mental endurance taught her to focus when distracted. Emotional endurance taught her to sit with difficult feelings. All of that transferred to her spiritual disciplines.

PRECEDING FEELING

"Be thou faithful unto death, and I will give thee a crown of life" (Revelation 2:10).

This commands faithfulness unto death, not faithfulness when you feel like it. Be faithful even when it costs you everything.

Hebrews 11:13–16 describes the heroes of faith.

"These all died in faith, not having received the promises, but having seen them afar off, and were persuaded of them, and embraced them, and confessed that they were strangers and pilgrims on the earth... But now they desire a better country, that is, an heavenly: wherefore God is not ashamed to be called their God: for he hath prepared for them a city" (Hebrews 11:13–16).

They died without receiving the promises. But they remained faithful anyway. That's spiritual endurance.

Moses chose reproach over Egypt's treasures (Hebrews 11:24–26). He endured suffering because he looked to the reward. He didn't quit when things got hard. He pressed through.

This is the call: faithfulness regardless of circumstances, obedience regardless of cost, endurance regardless of feelings.

And the payoff isn't always immediate. Sometimes you pray for years before breakthrough comes. You might obey for decades before you see fruit. Sometimes you endure trials that don't resolve until eternity.

But God honors endurance. And those who endure receive the crown of life.

PRACTICE PROMPT

❖ Commit to one spiritual discipline for thirty consecutive days, regardless of how it feels:
  - Daily prayer (even if just five minutes)
  - Daily Scripture reading (even if just one verse)

- Weekly church attendance (no skipping)
- ❖ Track two things:
    - How many days did you feel like doing it vs how many days you do it anyway?
    - What changes (if anything) by day thirty?
    - After thirty days, evaluate: Did endurance through dryness produce any fruit? What did you learn about your capacity?

Success Criteria

☐ You chose one specific spiritual discipline and practiced it for thirty consecutive days regardless of feeling.
☐ You tracked feeling vs. doing daily.
☐ You noted changes by day thirty.
☐ You evaluated what fruit emerged and what you learned about your capacity.

Troubleshooting

If you broke the streak, start over—it being thirty consecutive days matters.

If you consistently didn't feel like it but did it anyway, you're building exactly the muscle this exercise targets.

If nothing changed by day thirty, the fruit might be deeper than you can see yet. Ask someone close to you if they've noticed any shifts in you.

If thirty days feels overwhelming, start with seven days to build the habit, then extend to thirty.

If you felt like doing it most days, pick a more challenging discipline. You might be in a spiritually vibrant season.

HORMESIS

Strategic discomfort works because of a biological principle called hormesis: small doses of stress make the organism stronger.

The concept is simple: small doses of stress trigger adaptation. Large doses cause damage. No stress causes atrophy.

These are examples of hormesis:

- **Exercise:** Controlled stress on muscles triggers growth. No exercise makes muscles atrophy. Too much exercise, and injury occurs.
- **Fasting:** Controlled caloric restriction triggers metabolic adaptation. No fasting leads to metabolic inflexibility. Too much fasting causes starvation.
- **Cold exposure:** Controlled cold stress triggers thermogenic adaptation. No cold exposure leads to reduced resilience. Too much cold exposure causes hypothermia.
- **Mental challenge:** Controlled cognitive load strengthens focus. If there is no challenge, there will be cognitive decline. Too much challenge causes burnout.
- **Emotional sitting:** Controlled exposure to uncomfortable emotions (sitting long enough to name, analyze, and reframe) builds regulation capacity. Lack of emotional challenge develops avoidance and fragility. Too much emotional flooding causes trauma and dysregulation.

The dose matters. Strategic discomfort is about finding the zone where stress is high enough to trigger adaptation but low enough to avoid breakdown.

PRACTICE PROMPT

- ❖ Design your own strategic discomfort calendar for one week. Choose one controlled discomfort in each arena:

  - **Physical:** cold shower, extra mile, HIIT workout, or fasted training

  - **Mental:** difficult book, complex project, no phone for 4 hours

  - **Emotional:** honest conversation you've been avoiding, sitting with grief for 20 minutes

  - **Spiritual:** extended prayer, fasting, difficult passage study

❖ Do all four this week.

❖ Track how each one feels and what you learn.

❖ After the week, evaluate: Which was hardest? Which felt most beneficial?

❖ Design next week's calendar based on what you learned.

Success Criteria

☐ You designed a one-week calendar with one controlled discomfort in each of the four arenas.☐ You completed all four this week.

☐ You tracked how each felt and what you learned.

☐ You evaluated which was hardest and most beneficial. ☐ You designed next week's calendar.

Troubleshooting

If you only completed two or three out of four, that's still progress—but be honest about whether the barrier was time or avoidance.

If all four felt easy, you didn't choose true discomfort. Make them harder next week.

If one arena dominates in difficulty, that reveals where your endurance is weakest—spend extra time there.

If tracking felt like a chore, keep it to one sentence per discomfort.

If you didn't design next week's calendar, you're not treating this as an ongoing practice. The calendar isn't optional.

THE TRANSFER MECHANISM

Self-efficacy theory explains why endurance in one arena transfers to others.

Self-efficacy is your belief in your ability to succeed in specific situations. When you do a hard thing and succeed, you update your internal narrative: "I can do hard things."

That narrative generalizes. You don't just believe, "I can run thirty minutes without quitting." You start believing, "I can endure difficulty." That belief shows up everywhere.

Research on grit confirms this. People who develop perseverance in one domain (sports, academics, music) show increased perseverance in unrelated domains. The brain doesn't compartmentalize endurance. It builds a general bias toward persistence.

Every time you push through a quit urge (in any arena), you strengthen the endurance muscle globally.

PRACTICE PROMPT

❖ After your next endurance win (finishing a hard workout, completing a difficult mental task, staying in an uncomfortable emotion, persisting in a dry spiritual discipline), immediately ask, "Where else do I need this same capacity this week?"

❖ Then deliberately apply it within twenty-four hours.

❖ Track the following:

- The original endurance win
- Where you applied it
- Whether the transfer was successful
- How it felt different from doing it without the transfer

❖ Practice deliberate transfer weekly for a month. Notice if transfer becomes more automatic over time.

Success Criteria

☐ You identified your next endurance win.
☐ You immediately asked where else you need that capacity and applied it to a different arena within twenty-four hours.
☐ You tracked all four elements.
☐ You practiced this weekly for a month while observing if transfer becomes more automatic.

Troubleshooting

If you couldn't identify another area needing that capacity, you're not looking hard enough—every arena has challenges this week.

If you waited longer than twenty-four hours, the connection weakens. Move faster next time.

If the transfer wasn't successful, that's valuable data—some transfers work better than others. Keep experimenting.

If it felt exactly the same as without transfer, you didn't make the connection explicit enough. Before applying it, actually say out loud: "I endured X, so I can endure Y."

THE COMPOUNDING EFFECT

By week twelve, Alicia's life looks different.

Physically: She can run thirty-five minutes without quitting. Her resting heart rate dropped from seventy-eight to sixty-eight. Her body composition improved. She's stronger and more resilient. She walks up the stairs at work without getting winded. Her back pain decreased significantly.

Mentally: Alicia can focus deeply for two hours without degradation. Complex problems don't overwhelm her. Decision fatigue doesn't hit as hard. Her mind stays sharp under pressure. She's solving problems at work she used to avoid.

Emotionally: She can sit with difficult emotions for ten or more minutes without numbing or exploding. Her relationships improved. Marcus says she's more present, less defensive. Alicia's kids say she's less reactive. She's not perfect, but she's better.

Spiritually: She prays and reads Scripture daily, regardless of how it feels. She fasts weekly. Her faith is no longer feeling-dependent. God feels more real, even in the dry seasons. Alicia's serving at church again and having spiritual conversations with her kids.

But the most important change isn't in any single arena—it's in the whole system.

Alicia's physical endurance taught her to push through discomfort, which transferred to mental work. Her mental endurance taught her to stay focused under fatigue, which transferred to emotional regulation. Her emotional endurance taught her to sit with difficulty, which transferred to spiritual disciplines. And her spiritual endurance grounded everything else, giving her a transcendent purpose that motivated all the other work.

The arenas reinforce each other. Train one, and the others benefit. Train all four, and the effect compounds.

Alicia is not the same woman she was twelve weeks ago. She's not fragile anymore. She's not quitting as soon as things get hard. She's building endurance that lasts.

FOUR CRITICAL MISTAKES

Strategic discomfort is powerful, but it can be misapplied. Alicia made several mistakes along the way. Learn from them.

Mistake One: Confusing Stubbornness with Endurance
Week six: Alicia's knee starts hurting during her runs. It's sharp pain, not just discomfort. She ignores it. "Endurance means pushing through," she tells herself.

Week seven: Pain worsens. Alicia keeps running. "I'm building endurance. Winners don't quit."

Week eight: Alicia can barely walk. Her physical therapist's diagnosis is stress fracture developing in her tibia. Treatment: six weeks of no running, possibly eight if she doesn't rest properly.

Result: She is sidelined for six weeks because she confused stupidity with endurance.

The Difference

Endurance recognizes productive discomfort. Burning muscles (lactate buildup means she's being productive). Elevated heart rate (cardiovascular stress means she's being productive). Mental fatigue (cognitive challenge means she's being productive). Emotional discomfort (regulation practice means she's being productive).

Stubbornness ignores destructive pain. Sharp joint pain (injury developing) is destructive. Chest pain (cardiovascular emergency) is destructive. Dizziness/nausea (medical issue) is destructive. Inability to function (a breakdown) is destructive).

The Fix

Learn to distinguish signals. Productive discomfort says, "This is hard, but I can continue." Destructive pain says, "Something is wrong. I need to stop."

When in doubt, stop, assess, and get an expert opinion. Endurance without wisdom is just foolishness.

Mistake Two: Strategic Discomfort Without Recovery

Alicia got excited about strategic discomfort in week ten.

Monday: Cold shower + hard workout + difficult conversation with Marcus + extended fasting

Tuesday: Intense mental work + emotional confrontation with her boss + late-night work session

Wednesday: Long run + complex project + family tension + skipped meals

Thursday: HIIT workout + high-stress meeting + spiritual disciplines despite exhaustion

The Result (Week eleven)

Alicia experienced complete burnout + emotional emptiness + mentally fried + physical exhaustion + spiritual dryness. Alicia quit everything for a week. She went into full shutdown. Marcus found her crying in the bathroom. She said, "I can't do this anymore. I don't have anything left."

The Problem

It's all stress and no recovery. The body (and mind, heart, soul) adapts during rest, not during stress.

The Fix

Recovery is when adaptation happens. The formula is:

Stress + Recovery = Growth

Stress + Stress = Breakdown

Here's Alicia's corrected approach:
- Three to four days per week: strategic discomfort
- Two to three days per week: recovery (lighter activity, rest, enjoyment)
- One day per week: full rest (Sabbath principle)

Strategic discomfort requires strategic recovery.

Mistake Three: Using Endurance to Prove Worth

Week fifteen: Alicia starts tracking numbers obsessively.

She says, "I endured six hard things this week. Last week was only four. I need to do more."

She posts about her endurance wins on social media. She mentions her training in conversations. She starts comparing herself to others. "I ran thirty-five minutes today. Sarah at church can only run twenty minutes. I'm tougher."

Endurance becomes performance. Pride creeps in. She starts looking down on people who "quit too easily."

The problem

Endurance has become identity, not stewardship. It's about proving worth, not building capacity for service.

The Fix

"But I keep under my body, and bring it into subjection: lest that by any means, when I have preached to others, I myself should be a castaway" (1 Corinthians 9:27).

Paul disciplined his body for the sake of the gospel, not for personal glory.

"Let nothing be done through strife or vainglory; but in lowliness of mind let each esteem other better than themselves. Look not every man on his own things, but every man also on the things of others" (Philippians 2:3–4).

Endurance is for service, not superiority. You train so you can love better, serve longer, and carry others' burdens. The moment endurance becomes about proving you're better than someone else, you've missed the point.

Alicia's Corrected Conviction

"I'm building endurance so I can serve my family well, love Marcus patiently, disciple my kids effectively, and fulfill God's calling on my life. Not for pride, but for service. Not to prove worth, but to steward what God has given me. This is lifelong work. And it's worth it."

Mistake Four: Romanticizing Suffering (Staying in Harm)
Week eighteen: Alicia's friend Jessica hears about Alicia's endurance work. Jessica is in a toxic job. Her boss berates her daily. The environment is abusive. Jessica says, "I need to build endurance. I should stay and tough it out."

Alicia almost agrees. Then she realizes, that's not strategic discomfort. That's just harm.

The Difference

Strategic discomfort is chosen, controlled, and purposeful. You select the stressor. You control the dose. You have a clear purpose.

Harmful situations are unchosen, uncontrolled, and destructive. You didn't select the stressor. You can't control the dose. The purpose is unclear or absent.

Here are examples of strategic discomfort:

- Cold showers (chosen, controlled, build resilience)
- Hard workouts (chosen, controlled, build capacity)
- Difficult conversations (chosen, controlled, build relational health)
- Fasting (chosen, controlled, builds spiritual discipline)

Here are examples of harmful situations:

- Abusive relationships (unchosen harm, uncontrolled, destructive)
- Toxic work environments (unchosen stress, uncontrolled, destructive)
- Chronic sleep deprivation from overcommitment (uncontrolled, destructive)
- Self-imposed starvation or over-exercise (uncontrolled, destructive)

Ask three questions about any hardship:

- Did I choose this, or is it being imposed on me?
- Is this building my capacity or breaking me down?
- Is there a redemptive purpose, or is it just harm?

If it's unchosen, breaking you down, and lacking redemptive purpose, seek help. Make changes. Don't spiritualize abuse or harm.

PRACTICE PROMPT

Review the four mistakes. Which one are you most prone to?
1. Confusing endurance with stubbornness (ignoring injury signals)
2. Strategic discomfort without recovery (all stress, no rest)
3. Using endurance to prove worth (pride, comparison)
4. Romanticizing suffering (staying in harmful situations)

Write down one specific guardrail to prevent that mistake.

Here's an example guardrail: "If pain is sharp or worsening, I stop immediately and assess. Endurance doesn't mean ignoring injury."

Share your guardrail with your accountability partner. Ask them to call you out if they see you falling into that trap.

Success Criteria

☐ You reviewed all four mistakes, and identified which one you're most prone to.
☐ You wrote one specific guardrail to prevent it.
☐ You shared it with your accountability partner with permission for them to call you out.

Troubleshooting

If you think none of these applies to you, ask someone who knows you well which mistake they see you making. Often, we're blind to our own patterns.

If you wrote a guardrail, but it's vague ("I'll be more careful"), make it concrete with specific actions and triggers.

If you don't have an accountability partner, that itself is a problem—endurance work shouldn't be done in isolation. Find one this week.

If you shared the guardrail but your partner said, "Sure" without real engagement, pick someone who will actually hold you accountable.

MARKERS OF PROGRESS

Endurance-building is measurable. You don't have to guess whether it's working. Progress shows up in observable markers across all four arenas. Track your own data. Here's Alicia's as an example.

Physical Markers Week one vs Week twelve:
  Cardiovascular Endurance:

- Week one: Alicia can run ten minutes before wanting to quit.
- Week twelve: She can run thirty-five minutes before wanting to quit
- Measurable increase: 250%

Heart Rate at Same Effort:

- Week one: Alicia's heart rate is 175 at conversational pace.
- Week twelve: Her heart rate is 155 at the same pace.
- Measurable decrease: Her heart rate decreases by twenty bpm (stronger cardiovascular efficiency).

Recovery Time:

- Week one: Alicia needs seventy-two hours to recover from hard session.
- Week twelve: She needs thirty-six hours to recover from same session.
- Measurable improvement: She has a 50% faster recovery period.

Resting Heart Rate:

- Week one: Alicia's heart rate is seventy-eight bpm.
- Week twelve: Her heart rate is sixty-eight bpm.
- Measurable decrease: Alicia's heart rate decreased by ten bpm (improved cardiovascular fitness).

Mental Markers Week one vs Week twelve:

Sustained Focus Duration:

- Week one: Alicia can focus deeply for forty-five minutes before mental fatigue sets in.
- Week twelve: She can focus deeply for two hours before mental fatigue sets in.
- Measurable increase: Her focus increased by 166%.

Complex Problem-Solving Under Fatigue:

- Week one: Alicia cannot solve complex problems past hour three of work.
- Week twelve: She can solve complex problems (at reduced efficiency) up to hour five.
- Measurable improvement: She has increased her productive capacity by two hours.

Decision Quality Under Pressure:

- Week one: Alicia makes impulsive decisions when stressed.
- Week twelve: She can maintain analytical thinking under moderate stress.
- Measurable improvement: She has fewer decision regrets (Alicia tracks this).

Mental Fatigue Recovery:

- Week one: Alicia needs a full evening off after intense mental work.
- Week twelve: She can engage family meaningfully after intense mental work.
- Measurable improvement: She has faster cognitive recovery.

Emotional Markers Week one vs Week twelve:

Emotional Regulation Under Stress:

- Week one: Alicia snaps at kids within two minutes of

frustration.
- Week twelve: She can sit with frustration for ten or more minutes before responding.
- Measurable increase: She has five times the tolerance for discomfort.

Relationship Conflict Navigation:
- Week one: Alicia withdraws or attacks during tense conversations with Marcus.
- Week twelve: Alicia can stay present and engaged during difficult conversations.
- Measurable improvement: Marcus reports feeling heard and understood.

Emotional Recovery Time:
- Week one: Criticism at work ruins her entire day.
- Week twelve: Criticism at work impacts her for thirty to sixty minutes, then Alicia moves on.
- Measurable improvement: There is a ninety percent reduction in emotional hangover time.

Capacity for Difficult Emotions:
- Week one: Alicia avoids grief, anxiety, and anger whenever possible.
- Week twelve: She can sit with grief, anxiety, and anger without numbing herself.
- Measurable improvement: She is no longer dependent on distraction to regulate herself.

Spiritual Markers Week one vs Week twelve:

Consistency of Spiritual Disciplines:
- Week one: Alicia prays two to three times per week when she feels like it.
- Week twelve: She prays daily regardless of how it feels.
- Measurable increase: She increased her consistency by several days per week.

Scripture Engagement:
- Week one: Alicia reads Scripture sporadically (one to two times per week).
- Week twelve: She reads Scripture daily (seven times per week).
- Measurable increase: She has 350–700% more exposure to

Scripture.

Spiritual Resilience During Dry Seasons:
- Week one: Alicia quits spiritual disciplines when God feels distant.
- Week twelve: She maintains spiritual disciplines regardless of how she is feeling.
- Measurable improvement: Her faithfulness is independent of her feelings.

Fasting Discipline:
- Week one: Alicia never fasts.
- Week twelve: She fasts weekly from lunch.
- Measurable increase: She established a new discipline.

Integration Markers Week one vs Week twelve:

Cross-Arena Transfer:
- Week one: Weakness in one arena collapses others.
- Week twelve: Strength in one arena supports others.
- Measurable improvement: There is system-level resilience.

Capacity Under Compounding Stress:
- Week one: A single stressor (work deadline) impacts all arenas negatively.
- Week twelve: Alicia manages multiple stressors (work deadline + family tension + physical fatigue) without collapse.
- Measurable improvement: She can carry heavier loads simultaneously.

Overall Quit Point:

- Week one: Alicia quits when difficulty reaches 6/10 intensity.
- Week twelve: She pushes through difficulty up to 8/10 intensity before considering quitting.
- Measurable increase: Her tolerance threshold is thirty-three percent higher.

These markers are not about perfection. They're about progress. You're not comparing yourself to others. You're comparing yourself to yourself.

Track your markers quarterly. Write them down. Review

them. Celebrate progress. Identify weak spots. Adjust your protocol.

And remember: endurance-building is lifelong work. You don't "arrive." You keep training.

THE INVITATION

This chapter is not just theory. It is a strategic roadmap.

You are Alicia. Or you could be.

The question is: Will you stay comfortable and fragile, or will you choose strategic discomfort and build endurance that lasts?

The choice is yours, but the stakes are real.

Your family needs you to endure. Your church needs you to endure. The calling God has on your life requires endurance you may not currently have.

So start—today.

Choose one act of strategic discomfort this week. Physical options include cold showers, extra miles, or workouts that push your limits. Mental challenges might involve difficult reading, complex projects, or sustained focus sessions. Emotional work could mean initiating an honest conversation, sitting with grief, or tolerating intensity without numbing yourself. Spiritual disciplines might include extended prayer, fasting, or studying difficult passages.

Do it. Track it. Repeat it.

Build the endurance muscle. Do it one rep at a time, one week at a time, and one arena at a time. Watch what happens when your quit point moves.

"I can do all things through Christ which strengtheneth me"

(Philippians 4:13).

That's the foundation. It's not self-reliance or personal toughness. It's Christ's strength working through disciplined preparation.

CHAPTER SIX
THE RELATIONAL CROSS

A HOUSE OF WELLNESS

I'd been coaching people for over a decade. I'd seen the pattern: the clients who reached their goals had people in their corner. The ones who struggled were isolated, even when they were surrounded by people. I'd researched the science. Strong relationships increase survival by fifty percent. Isolation is as deadly as smoking fifteen cigarettes a day. I knew this intellectually.

Halfway through a podcast, I hit pause. Two pastors were breaking down how to think about your relationships using a cross: horizontal for friendships, vertical for mentorship. The idea stuck.

But I'd never actually mapped my own relational cross.

I grabbed a pen and sketched it out. I drew a cross and started filling in names. The horizontal line was for friends. The vertical line was for people above me who were pouring into me and people below me that I was investing in. What I saw forced me to sit with some uncomfortable truths.

Some people were way too close. I was treating them like my inner circle when they should've been further out. Others weren't close enough. People who deserved more from me weren't getting it because I was spread too thin. But the biggest gap was above me. The vertical line where mentors should be was basically empty.

At the time of this writing, I'm in my forties. I coach people for a living. I pour into others constantly. That part of the cross is fine. But who's pouring into me? Whom am I sitting with to get perspective from someone ten years ahead? Nobody. And it's not pride. It's trust. I don't trust easily. Never have. But that doesn't change the fact that the gap is real, and it's costing me.

Here's what else hit me while staring at that sketch: the pastors never mentioned the center. They just talked about the horizontal and vertical. But the center matters. That's where you are. That's where God is. For me, that's where my wife is, too, because we're one. If the center is cracked, the whole cross collapses.

I don't have a lot of relationships. There's my wife, and a handful of others scattered across that cross. That's it. Looking at that drawing forced me to admit: this structure is thin. Functional, but thin. It was one crisis away from buckling because the support wasn't there.

I'm working on it now, trying to figure out who I can actually trust above me. I'm adjusting who gets access to what level and building what should've been built years ago.

The Cost of Ignoring the Relational Cross

That's why this chapter exists—not because I have it figured out but because I've lived the cost of ignoring it. You can have a sound heart, sharp mind, strong body, and an anchored soul and still collapse if the relational structure isn't there to hold you up when life gets hard.

Out of all the chapters, this one's different. This is about the people around you, where they belong, and why it matters more than you think.

The four main chapters focused on stewarding yourself: training your heart, sharpening your mind, strengthening your body, and watering your soul. But the Great Commandment doesn't end there. Love the Lord your God with all your heart, soul, mind, and strength. Then Love your neighbor as yourself. The four arenas prepare you. Relationships are where that preparation gets tested, expressed, and multiplied.

Here's the working definition: **healthy relationships are mutual connections that strengthen your capacity to love God and serve others.** They provide accountability, encouragement, correction, and companionship.

A sound heart steadies your words when conflict hits, a sound mind helps you discern who belongs where on your cross. A strong body extends your capacity to show up consistently instead of burning out, and a strong soul anchors your love in something deeper than emotion or convenience.

But none of that happens automatically. You need structure, a framework. It needs to be something biblical that shows you who belongs where, how close they should be, and how much weight each relationship should carry.

That's what the relational cross gives you.

Jesus modeled this. He had the three: Peter, James, John. Then the twelve. Then the seventy-two. Then the crowds. He had different circles with different levels of access. Each involved different amounts of investment. He knew exactly who belonged where. He stewarded relational intensity with precision.

This chapter maps that same structure for your life. You'll learn how to build a cross that actually bears weight. You'll see how to avoid the pitfalls that collapse connection and how to love others well by first stewarding yourself well.

You can have a sound heart, sharp mind, strong body, and an anchored soul and still collapse if the relational structure isn't there when life gets hard. That's what this chapter fixes.

THE RELATIONAL CROSS AS A MAP

Jesus gave us the cross as the blueprint.

"If anyone would come after me, let him deny himself and take up his cross daily and follow me" (Luke 9:23).

He wasn't talking about substitution. He already bore that cross for our salvation once for all. This is about discipleship, surrender, and daily stewardship.

The cross works as a relational framework. Picture it: you're at the center. The horizontal line stretches left and right, representing reciprocal friendships, the people who walk alongside you. The vertical line stretches up and down, representing mentorship.

Above you are those pouring wisdom and correction into your life. Below you are those you're investing in, discipling, and pouring into.

Proximity to the center determines intensity. The closer someone is to you at the center, the more weight that relationship carries, the more time it requires, the more influence it has. Further out has less weight, less intensity, but is still valuable. Jesus had Peter, James, and John close. Then the twelve. Then the seventy-two. Then the crowds. Each circle served a purpose. Each required different investment.

Science backs it up. Strong relational ties reduce stress, improve immunity, and literally extend your life. Weak or absent ties accelerate decline. The cross is the model. Stewardship of relationships is the call.

THE LANGUAGE OF CONNECTION

Scripture doesn't speak about relationships in vague, sentimental terms. It uses precise language that reveals what God designed connection to be.

Koinonia: Partnership in Purpose

The Greek word *koinonia* (κοινωνία) appears twenty times in the New Testament. It's often translated "fellowship," but that translation is too weak. *Koinonia* means partnership, participation, sharing in common. It's not casual socializing. It's joint ownership of a mission.

Acts 2:42 describes the early church:

"They devoted themselves to the apostles' teaching and to koinonia, to the breaking of bread and to prayer" (Acts 2:42).

This wasn't a book club. This was people pooling resources, sharing burdens, and living intertwined lives for a common purpose.

When Paul writes to Philemon about Onesimus, he calls him a "partner" (*koinonos*), someone who shares in the work. That's the quality Scripture demands from meaningful relationships: mutual investment, shared sacrifice, common purpose.

Hesed: Covenant Love That Endures

The Hebrew word *hesed* is one of the richest words in Scripture. It appears over 240 times in the Old Testament. It's often translated "steadfast love," "lovingkindness," or "mercy," but none of those capture it fully.

Hesed is covenant loyalty. It's the love that refuses to quit even when circumstances change. It's Ruth saying to Naomi, in Ruth 1:16, "Where you go I will go, and where you stay I will stay." It's Jonathan protecting David even when it cost him the throne. It's God's promise to Abraham that holds across generations.

This is what covenant relationships require: faithfulness across time and hardship. It's not convenience-based connection that evaporates under pressure but loyalty that lasts. *Hesed* doesn't walk away when things get hard. It digs in deeper.

Jesus' Relational Model: The Circles of Intimacy

Jesus didn't treat all relationships the same. He had concentric circles of connection, each with different levels of access and investment.

His innermost circle was the three: Peter, James, and John. They were invited to the Mount of Transfiguration (Matthew 17:1), to Gethsemane (Matthew 26:37), to witness the raising of Jairus' daughter (Mark 5:37). They saw him at his most vulnerable, most raw, most human. Then came the twelve disciples. He taught them privately, corrected them, ate with them, and sent them out. They traveled, lived, and learned together. The relationship was intimate but broader than the three. Beyond that were the seventy-two, sent out in pairs to prepare towns (Luke 10:1). These were ministry partners, still personally commissioned but at a greater relational distance. Then the crowds. He taught, healed, and fed them. He also withdrew from them to pray (Luke 5:16). The crowds received teaching and miracles but not intimacy.

Finally, he had time alone with the Father: in the early mornings (Mark 1:35), all-night prayer (Luke 6:12), and the wilderness (Matthew 4:1). Solitude with God anchored everything else.

Notice the pattern: Jesus had deep investment with a few, wider connection with many, and protected time alone with God. He didn't try to be everything to everyone. He stewarded relational intensity with precision.

THE BIOLOGY OF BELONGING

Scripture told us relationships matter. Modern science confirms exactly how they matter, down to the cellular level.

Back in 2010, researchers reviewed 148 studies involving over 308,000 people. The finding was stark: **strong social relationships increase your likelihood of survival by fifty percent.** Not five percent. Fifty. That's comparable to quitting smoking. It exceeds the impact of obesity and physical inactivity. Point blank, connection keeps you alive longer.

Here's how it works in your body:

Cortisol drops when you're connected. When you're in supportive relationships, your stress hormone levels literally decrease. Your body relaxes at a chemical level. Chronic loneliness keeps cortisol elevated, which suppresses immune function, raises blood pressure, and accelerates cognitive decline. Your body treats isolation like a threat.

Oxytocin releases during safe connection. Physical touch, emotional safety, and trust trigger oxytocin, the bonding hormone. Oxytocin reduces anxiety, lowers heart rate, and promotes healing. That's why hugging a friend after bad news actually helps. It's not just sentiment. It's biochemistry.

Inflammation increases when you're isolated. Social isolation increases inflammatory markers like C-reactive protein and interleukin-6. Chronic inflammation is linked to heart disease, diabetes, cancer, and Alzheimer's. Loneliness inflames. Connection heals.

Your nervous system responds to relational safety. Stephen Porges' research shows that safe relationships activate the ventral vagal complex, which regulates heart rate, breathing, and digestion. When you feel safe with someone, your body literally shifts into rest-and-digest mode. Toxic relationships trigger a fight-or-flight response. Your body knows the difference.

John Cacioppo's research at the University of Chicago found that loneliness is as dangerous to health as smoking fifteen cigarettes a day. Isolated people have higher blood pressure, a weakened immune response, increased inflammation, disrupted sleep, accelerated cognitive decline, and higher rates of depression and anxiety.

This isn't about being an introvert or extrovert but about isolation versus connection. You can be alone and not lonely if you have strong bonds. You can be surrounded by people and desperately lonely if the connections are shallow or toxic. Your body doesn't care about your social media follower count. It cares about whether you have real relationships where you feel known, safe, and connected.

PRACTICE PROMPT—PART 1

This should take you about ten to fifteen minutes.

- ❖ Map your current relational cross on paper. Draw a cross. Put yourself at the center. On the horizontal line, write the names of your closest friends. On the vertical line above, write mentors or those who pour into you. Below, write those you're pouring into. In the outer areas, write acquaintances and broader connections.

- ❖ Look at what you've drawn. Where are the gaps? Where is there imbalance? Is the horizontal line empty? Is the vertical line one-sided? Are you isolated at the center?

- ❖ Write one specific action you'll take this week to strengthen it.

Success Criteria

☐ You drew your *actual* relational cross (not an idealized version).

☐ You identified at least one specific gap or imbalance.

☐ You wrote down one concrete action to address it (not "Be better at friendships" but "Text John to schedule coffee this week").

☐ You followed through within seven days.

Troubleshooting

If your cross looks perfectly balanced, you're either unusually healthy relationally or you're lying to yourself. Ask your spouse or a close friend to look at it and tell you what they see.

If you identified a gap but didn't take action within seven days, your relational issues are theoretical to you, not urgent. Ask yourself what the cost of continuing as you are is.

If you can't identify any gaps, you might be so disconnected that you can't see the isolation. That's the most dangerous place to be.

GIVING WHAT YOU DO NOT HAVE

The relational cross begins at the center with you in relationship with God. This is the foundation. Jesus modeled this pattern throughout his ministry. He withdrew regularly to pray alone (Luke 5:16). He prayed in the early mornings (Mark 1:35) and had all-night prayer sessions (Luke 6:12) and extended time in the wilderness (Matthew 4:1). His relationship with the Father was the source from which everything else flowed. You cannot give what you do not have.

For those who are married, the center includes your spouse. Genesis 2:24 says, "Therefore a man shall leave his father and his mother and hold fast to his wife, and they shall become one flesh." Two become one. This isn't a metaphor. It's the nature of covenant marriage.

Ephesians reinforces this:

"Husbands should love their wives as their own bodies. He who loves his wife loves himself. For no one ever hated his own flesh, but nourishes and cherishes it" (Ephesians 5:28–29).

Centers

The center for a married person is God + you + your spouse as one unit. For a single person, the center is God + you. Both require the same stewardship: a sound heart, sound mind, strong body, and a strong soul that is anchored in relationship with God. Marriage adds a unique dimension. Your spouse isn't on the horizontal axis with friends. Your spouse is at the center with you because you are one flesh.

This changes how you steward the center. A single person can focus entirely on their own formation in relationship with God. A married person must steward their own formation while simultaneously stewarding the covenant union. You can't neglect yourself and expect to love your spouse well. You can't neglect your spouse and claim you're stewarding the center. Both require attention.

When Jesus said to love your neighbor as yourself, he was pointing to a prerequisite: you must be anchored in God's love for you before you can genuinely love yourself. Only then can you extend that love outward to others. For married people, your spouse is not your neighbor. Your spouse is yourself. "The two shall become one flesh." You are to love your spouse as your own body, which means stewarding their heart, mind, body, and soul matters as much as stewarding your own.

This is why The SCAL Method starts with individual formation before moving to relational integration. A sound heart stabilizes your emotional presence in your marriage and other relationships. Having a sound mind means that your discernment about whom to invest in and when to set boundaries is sharp. A strong body extends your capacity to show up consistently for your spouse and others. A strong soul, rooted in communion with God, anchors your purpose so relationships *serve* the mission instead of *becoming* the mission.

Here's the tension: you cannot steward the center in isolation from other people beyond your spouse. The cross is inherently relational. Even in marriage, you need friendships, mentors, and those you invest in. You need others to hold you accountable, to sharpen you, to correct you, to encourage you. First Corinthians 12 describes the body of Christ as interconnected parts. The eye cannot say to the hand, "I don't need you." You need the horizontal and vertical relationships to steward the center well, but the center must be strong enough to support those relationships.

Jesus stewarded his connection with the Father, which gave him the strength to pour into the twelve, the seventy-two, and the crowds. The center held because he protected it. When the center was full, he could give without depletion.

Example: Ben's Center

Ben is thirty-eight. He's a senior engineer at a tech company. He has been married for eleven years to Sarah. Ben is the father of two boys, ages eight and five. He goes to church most Sundays and volunteers in the community.

On paper, Ben's life looks solid, but Ben's center is cracking, and it's affecting his marriage.

Ben hasn't taken a full day off in eight months. He sleeps five hours a night. His workouts stopped six months ago. He prays occasionally but feels nothing. When he does pray, it's rushed, distracted, perfunctory. "God, bless this day. Help me get through it. Amen." He prays for thirty seconds, then he's checking his phone.

Ben's relationship with God has become transactional rather than relational. He goes to church out of habit not hunger. He reads his Bible sporadically, skimming verses without letting them penetrate. His spiritual life is on autopilot, and the autopilot is failing.

His heart is a mess: he feels resentment toward his boss, anxiety about money, and guilt about not being more present with his kids. Ben hasn't processed any of these emotions. He just pushes them down and keeps moving. His mind is foggy from exhaustion. He can't focus during meetings and forgets conversations. His body is twenty-five pounds overweight and his back hurts constantly. His soul feels dry, disconnected, going through motions without meaning.

Sarah feels it. She's tried to reach him. "Ben, talk to me. What's going on?"

He deflects. "I'm fine. Just busy. Work's crazy right now." But it's been "crazy" for two years.

She knows he's not fine. She can see the exhaustion, the distance, the withdrawal. She's lonely in her own marriage because Ben is physically present but emotionally absent.

The center isn't just weak. It's fractured. Ben is neglecting his relationship with God, neglecting his own heart, mind, body, and soul; as a result, he's neglecting Sarah. He tells himself he's working hard for his family, providing for them, sacrificing for them. But he's not present with them. He's going through the motions while internally collapsing.

Sarah has tried to talk about it. She's suggested counseling.

Ben brushed it off. "We don't need counseling. We're fine." But they're not fine. The distance is growing. The resentment is building. Ben is too exhausted to engage emotionally, and Sarah is tired of feeling like she's married to a ghost.

Here's what Ben doesn't see: when he neglects himself, he's also neglecting Sarah. They are one flesh. When he lets his health deteriorate, it affects her. When he refuses to process his emotions, she absorbs the fallout. When his soul is dry, their marriage suffers. You cannot steward the center alone in a marriage. You steward it together, or it crumbles together.

The center isn't holding. And until Ben addresses his relationship with God and his stewardship of heart, mind, body, and soul, and until he reconnects with Sarah as one flesh instead of two people living parallel lives, no amount of external activity will fix what's breaking internally.

PRACTICE PROMPT—PART 1

❖ Assess the strength of your center honestly. Rate yourself 1–10 in these areas:
  - **Relationship with God:** How connected, not just dutiful, is your prayer life and time in Scripture?
  - **Heart:** How well are you regulating emotions rather than suppressing or being ruled by them?
  - Mind: How clear is your thinking? Are you sharp or foggy?
  - **Body:** How consistently are you training, sleeping, and eating well?
  - **Soul:** How anchored do you feel in purpose and peace?
  - **Marriage (if applicable):** How emotionally present and engaged are you with your spouse?

❖ Identify your lowest score. Write down one specific action you'll take this week to strengthen that area.

Success Criteria

☐ You rated all areas honestly (not aspirationally).☐ You identified your weakest area and wrote one concrete action to address it (not "Pray more" but "Pray for ten minutes every morning before checking my phone").

☐ You executed that action at least five out of seven days.

☐ If you're married, you also had one honest conversation with your spouse about your assessment.

Troubleshooting

If everything scored eight or above, you're either exceptionally healthy or lying to yourself. Ask your spouse or close friend to rate you in these areas and compare notes. If you identified the weakness but didn't follow through five days, your stated priorities don't match your actual priorities.

The center won't strengthen by accident—it requires deliberate daily choices. If your relationship with God scored lowest and you're avoiding addressing it, ask yourself why. What are you afraid of finding if you slow down and actually connect with Him? If you're married and your marriage scored lowest but you didn't have an honest conversation with your spouse, you're avoiding the vulnerability required for covenant. Start there.

THE HORIZONTAL AXIS

The horizontal line of the cross represents reciprocal relationships, friendships where the give and take flows both directions. These are the people who walk beside you, not above or below, but alongside. They're your peers, your companions, the ones who share the journey with you.

Scripture shows us what covenant friendship looks like through Jonathan and David. First Samuel 18:1 says Jonathan's soul was knit to David's soul, and Jonathan loved him as his own soul. This acquaintance wasn't casual. It was covenant. Jonathan gave David his robe, his armor, his sword, his bow, and his belt. He stripped himself of the symbols of his own status and shared them with his friend. Later, when Saul tried to kill David, Jonathan protected him even though it cost Jonathan the throne (1 Samuel 20). That's *hesed* in action. Covenant loyalty refuses to quit when the cost gets high.

Horizontal friendships operate at different intensities based on proximity to the center. Not every friend needs to be a Jonathan-level friendship. Jesus had the three, the twelve, the seventy-two, and the crowds. Each circle served a purpose. The key is having at least some covenant-level friendships close to the center.

The Three Levels of Horizontal Connection

Covenant Level (Close to Center)

These are the two to five people who know you deeply. They've seen you at your worst and stayed. You can call them at 2AM. You share real struggles, not just surface updates. These relationships require mutual vulnerability, consistent presence, and willingness to speak hard truth in love.

"Iron sharpens iron, and one man sharpens another" (Proverbs 27:17).

That sharpening happens in covenant friendships. It's not always comfortable, but it's essential.

These friendships carry weight. They require time, energy, and emotional investment. You can't have fifty covenant-level friends. The human brain and the person's schedule won't support it. You need at least one or two. Without them, you're isolated at the center even if you're surrounded by people.

Middle Circle (Moderate Distance)

These are friends you see regularly, share common interests with, and genuinely enjoy. You might work together, serve together in ministry, train together at the gym, or share a hobby. The relationship is real but not as deep as covenant level. You know each other well enough to have meaningful conversation, but you're not processing the darkest struggles together.

These friendships provide community, encouragement, and shared activity. They buffer loneliness and create social connection. Galatians 6:10 says to do good to everyone, especially those of the household of faith. The middle circle is where much of that "doing good" happens. You serve together, celebrate together, and support each other in practical ways.

Outer Circle (Greater Distance)

These are acquaintances—people you know by name, neighbors you wave to, parents at your kids' school, and colleagues you chat with occasionally. The connection is friendly but not deep. These relationships still matter.

Mark Granovetter's research on "the strength of weak ties" shows that casual acquaintances often provide unique opportunities, information, and resources that close friends don't. A job lead might come from someone in your outer circle. You might receive a helpful introduction or a perspective you hadn't considered.

The outer circle also serves as the pool from which deeper friendships can develop. Most covenant friendships start as acquaintances, then move closer over time through shared experience and intentional investment.

Example: Ben's Horizontal Relationships

Ben's horizontal line is barren. He has exactly zero covenant friendships. His best friend from college moved across the country five years ago. They text occasionally but haven't had a real conversation in two years. There's no one Ben can call at 2 AM if everything falls apart. No one who knows what's actually going on inside him.

In the middle circle, Ben has work colleagues he eats lunch with. They talk about projects, sports, and weekend plans. It's all surface-level stuff. If Ben stopped showing up tomorrow, they'd notice for a week, then move on. These are acquaintances masquerading as friends.

Ben's outer circle includes guys from church he nods at on Sundays, neighbors he waves to, and parents from his kids' school. They are friendly, polite, and completely disconnected from anything real.

The horizontal line of Ben's cross is essentially empty. He has no reciprocal friendships where burdens are shared, truth is spoken, and presence is consistent. When work gets stressful, he has no one to process with. When his marriage hits friction, he withdraws instead of seeking counsel. The isolation compounds the stress, and the stress deepens the isolation.

What Kills Horizontal Friendships

Friendships don't usually die from dramatic conflict. They die slowly from neglect. Three patterns destroy horizontal relationships faster than anything else.

Busyness as Default Excuse

I'm too busy" becomes the go-to response. Weeks become months. Months become years. You tell yourself you'll reconnect when things calm down, but things never calm down. Meanwhile, the friendship atrophies. Proverbs 18:24 says there is a friend who sticks closer than a brother, but that sticking requires showing up. Busyness that chronically displaces friendship reveals what you actually prioritize.

Refusal to Be Vulnerable

You keep conversations surface-level. Everything's "fine." You're "busy but good." Meanwhile, you're drowning internally, but you'd rather maintain the image than admit struggle. This kills covenant-level friendship because covenant requires honesty. If you won't let people in, they can't walk with you. Galatians 6:2 says to bear one another's burdens, but you can't bear what isn't shared.

Scorekeeping Instead of Grace

You track who called last, who initiated last, who gave more effort. When it feels unbalanced, you pull back. "I'm not going to be the only one trying." Maybe the imbalance is real. Maybe the other person is genuinely checked out.

Often scorekeeping poisons what could be restored through honest conversation. You just withdraw instead of saying, "I've felt distant from you lately. Can we talk?" The friendship dies in silence.

THE VERTICAL AXIS

Theverticallineofthecrossrepresentsnonreciprocalrelationships. Above you are mentors, those pouring wisdom, correction, and perspective into your life. Below you are those you're investing in, pouring into, and discipling. These relationships aren't equal in the way horizontal friendships are. One person gives, the other receives. That's the design.

Above: Those Who Pour Into You

Mentorship is not friendship. A mentor is not your peer. A mentor is someone further along the path who has walked where you're walking and can guide you through terrain you haven't navigated yet. Hebrews says,

"Remember your leaders, those who spoke to you the word of God. Consider the outcome of their way of life, and imitate their faith" (Hebrews 13:7).

Good mentors do three things:

- ask hard questions you're avoiding
- challenge assumptions you're clinging to
- see patterns you can't see because you're too close

A mentor doesn't need to be perfect. They need to be further ahead than you in the specific area where you need guidance. Have they been married thirty years? They can mentor you on marriage. Have they built a business? They can mentor you on entrepreneurship. Did they walk through grief? They can mentor you through loss.

Most people resist seeking mentors because it requires admitting you don't have it figured out. It feels vulnerable to ask for help. But Scripture tells us to.

"Whoever walks with the wise becomes wise, but the companion of fools will suffer harm" (Proverbs 13:20).

You become like the people you spend time with. Choose mentors who have what you want: character, wisdom, and other spiritual fruit.

Below: Those You Pour Into

Investment below is generativity, the drive to contribute to future generations. Erikson called this a core developmental task of adulthood. Paul modeled it to Timothy.

"What you have heard from me in the presence of many witnesses entrust to faithful men, who will be able to teach others also" (2 Timothy 2:2).

Four generations are in one verse: Paul, Timothy, faithful men, and others. The knowledge went from Paul to Timothy, Timothy to faithful men, then from the faithful men to others.

Pouring into others forces you to clarify what you believe. You can't disciple someone else if you're unclear yourself. It also keeps you humble. You're reminded how hard the basics are. You see your own failures reflected in someone else's struggles. You're confronted with how much grace you needed when you were where they are now.

Investment below doesn't require a formal title or credentials. You don't need to be ordained to mentor a younger believer. You don't need a degree to help someone navigate a challenge you've already faced. All that is needed is willingness to share what you've learned and presence to walk with them through it.

Example: Ben's Vertical Relationships

Ben has no mentor. There is no one above him pouring wisdom, correction, or perspective into his life. He had a boss he respected years ago, but that guy retired. His father passed away when Ben was twenty-two, and they weren't close anyway. His pastor is kind but overextended; Ben's never had a one-on-one conversation with him beyond pleasantries.

Ben tells himself he doesn't need a mentor. He's almost forty. He's got things figured out. Except he doesn't. His marriage is strained, and he doesn't know how to fix it. His career has plateaued, and he's not sure what's next. His spiritual life feels dry, and he doesn't know how to reconnect. These are exactly the areas where someone ten years ahead could offer perspective, but Ben's pride keeps him from asking for help.

Below Ben, there's no one he's investing in, either. He doesn't disciple anyone. He doesn't mentor a younger guy at work or church. He's not pouring into his sons beyond basic parenting: help with homework, drive to soccer, make sure they brush their teeth. He's managing their behavior but not forming their character. There's no intentional discipleship happening.

The vertical axis is as empty as the horizontal. Ben stands alone at the center, disconnected above and below, isolated on all sides.

What Kills Vertical Relationships

Pride kills mentorship above. You tell yourself you don't need help. You've made it this far on your own. Asking for guidance feels like admitting weakness. So you keep pushing forward without wisdom from those who've gone before. First Corinthians 3:5–7 reminds us that Paul planted, Apollos watered, but God gave the growth. You're part of a relay, not the whole race. Receive the baton from those ahead.

Impatience kills investment below. Discipleship is slow. People don't change overnight. You pour in for months and see minimal fruit. You get frustrated and pull back, but spiritual formation works on God's timeline, not yours. You're planting and watering. God gives the growth. Your job is faithfulness, not results.

Hero worship distorts mentorship. You elevate your mentor to guru status. You want them to be perfect, to have all the answers, to never disappoint. When they inevitably fail or fall short, you're crushed. Galatians 1:10 warns against seeking to please man rather than God. Learn from mentors, but don't worship them. They're human, flawed, still growing. Take what's good. Discern what's useful. Leave what's not.

PRACTICE PROMPT—PART 2

❖ **Week 1:** Identify one person you could invest in (below) and one person you could learn from (above). Don't reach out yet. Just observe. Who's asking questions you could help answer? Who has walked a path you're on now?

❖ **Week 2:** Reach out to one of them. For the person below, offer to meet for coffee and share what you've learned in an area they're navigating. For the person above, ask if they'd be willing to meet occasionally to offer perspective on a specific challenge you're facing.

Success Criteria

☐ You identified specific people (with names, not categories like "someone at church").
☐ You reached out to at least one within two weeks.
☐ You scheduled a meeting and actually showed up for it.

Troubleshooting

If you can't identify anyone to invest in, you're not paying attention to the people around you. Look at your church, workplace, and neighborhood. Someone younger is struggling with something you've already navigated.

If you can't identify anyone above you, your pride is blocking your vision. Find someone ten years ahead in an area you want to grow.

If you identified people but didn't reach out, fear is stopping you. It may be fear of being rejected, looking needy, or committing. Name the fear, then reach out anyway. The worst they can say is no.

INTENSITY AND DISTANCE

Not all relationships should carry the same weight. Proximity to the center determines intensity. The closer someone is to the center of your cross, the more relational energy they require and the more influence they have on your life.

Jesus modeled this. Peter, James, and John were closer than the other nine disciples. The twelve were closer than the seventy-two. The seventy-two were closer than the crowds. Jesus didn't treat everyone the same. He stewarded relational intensity with precision.

This isn't favoritism. It's wisdom. You have limited time,

emotional energy, and capacity. Trying to invest equally in everyone spreads you so thin that no relationship gets what it needs. Instead, you must discern: Who is covenant-level? Who is middle circle? Who is outer circle? And steward each level appropriately.

Proverbs warns us about this.

"Let your foot be seldom in your neighbor's house, lest he have his fill of you and hate you" (Proverbs 25:17).

Even good relationships can be damaged by too much proximity without appropriate boundaries. Intensity must match the level of commitment and mutual investment. Forcing intimacy where covenant doesn't exist creates resentment. Withholding presence where covenant does exist creates abandonment.

The Danger of Misplaced Intensity

When you give covenant-level energy to someone who's only in the middle or outer circle, you drain yourself without building anything sustainable. They didn't sign up for that level of investment. You're pouring into someone who isn't equipped or willing to reciprocate. The relationship becomes one-sided, exhausting, eventually toxic.

The reverse is also destructive. When you treat covenant-level people like acquaintances, offering surface-level engagement when they need depth, they feel abandoned. Your spouse, your closest friends, your covenant relationships require consistent presence, vulnerability, and investment. If you're giving them leftovers while pouring energy into shallow connections, the most important relationships in your life will deteriorate.

"Whoever walks with the wise becomes wise, but the companion of fools will suffer harm" (Proverbs 13:20).

You become like the people closest to you. Choose wisely who occupies the inner circle. Not everyone deserves access to the center. Not everyone has earned the right to speak into your life at that level. Distance isn't rejection. It's discernment.

Practical Guardrails

Ask yourself three questions about each relationship:

- **Does this relationship make me more like Christ or less?**
- **Is this relationship reciprocal or one-sided?**
- **Does this person sharpen me or dull me?**

Does this relationship make me more like Christ or less? First Corinthians 15:33 warns that bad company corrupts good morals. If a relationship consistently pulls you away from God, your purpose, or health and wholeness, then it needs distance. It's not cruelty or cutting someone off without explanation. It is deliberate distance to protect what God is building in you.

Is this relationship reciprocal or one-sided? Covenant friendships require mutual investment. If you're always initiating, giving, and carrying the weight while the other person shows up when it's convenient, that's not covenant. That's acquaintance pretending to be friendship. Move it to the appropriate circle.

Does this person sharpen me or dull me? Proverbs 27:17 says iron sharpens iron. Sharpening requires friction. It's not always comfortable. There's a difference between the discomfort of being challenged to grow and the exhaustion of managing someone's chaos. Sharpening produces clarity. Chaos produces fog. Know the difference.

HOW RELATIONSHIPS INTEGRATE

Relationships don't exist in isolation from the four arenas. They're woven through all of them, amplifying or undermining each one.

Sound Heart

A sound heart regulates emotions, which stabilizes your presence in relationships. When your heart is trained, you don't lash out in anger, withdraw in fear, or manipulate through guilt. You can receive correction without defensiveness. You can give feedback without cruelty. You can sit with someone in their pain without trying to fix it immediately.

Reciprocally, healthy relationships steady the heart. When you're in covenant friendships where you can name emotions honestly without judgment and process grief, anger, or fear with people who won't abandon you, your nervous system learns safety. Cortisol drops. Oxytocin rises. The heart stabilizes because you're not carrying everything alone.

Toxic relationships wreck the heart. Constant criticism keeps you in sympathetic nervous system overdrive. Manipulation trains you to suppress emotions in order to keep the peace. Abandonment teaches you that vulnerability leads to rejection.

A sound heart requires healthy relational soil to grow in.

Sound Mind

A sound mind thinks clearly, discerns well, and resists manipulation. Wise mentors sharpen your thinking by asking questions you haven't considered, challenging assumptions you're clinging to, and providing perspective you can't see from where you stand.

"Oil and perfume make the heart glad, and the sweetness of a friend comes from his earnest counsel" (Proverbs 27:9).

Relationships also test your thinking. When you articulate to someone else what you believe, you're forced to clarify.

Fuzzy thinking gets exposed in conversation. Iron sharpens iron. Your mind gets sharper when people who think well challenge you to think better.

But relationships can also cloud the mind. When you surround yourself with people who never question you, who affirm everything you say, who tell you what you want to hear instead of what you need to hear, your thinking gets lazy.

Proverbs warns us about this.

"The way of a fool is right in his own eyes, but a wise man listens to advice" (Proverbs 12:15).

Choose relationships that sharpen, not flatter.

Strong Body

Physical training is easier when you're not doing it alone. Accountability partners show up even when motivation fades. Training partners push you harder than you'd push yourself.

Community makes consistency sustainable.

Research shows that social support significantly improves adherence to exercise programs. You're more likely to keep training if someone else is counting on you to show up. If the people around you eat well, you're more likely to eat well, too. You're more likely to prioritize sleep if your spouse values rest.

The reverse is also true. If your closest relationships normalize sedentary living, poor nutrition, and chronic exhaustion, you'll drift toward those patterns. Your body responds to the culture of your relational environment.

Strong Soul

Spiritual formation happens in community.

"Let us consider how to stir up one another to love and good works, not neglecting to meet together, as is the habit of some, but encouraging one another" (Hebrews 10:24–25).

You need other believers to sharpen your faith, to remind you of truth when you forget, to pray for you when you're weak, to call you back when you drift.

Mentors model what mature faith looks like. You see how they handle suffering, love difficult people, and stay faithful over decades. Investment below forces you to articulate what you believe. Discipling someone else keeps your own faith active and clear.

But spiritual formation also requires solitude. You need time alone with God that time with others can't replace. Jesus withdrew regularly. So must you. Relationships support the soul, but they don't substitute for direct communion with God.

Example: Ben's Rebuilt Cross

We've seen Ben's cracked center. We've seen his empty horizontal and vertical axes. Now let's see what happens when Ben rebuilds the cross.

Ben's Center Rebuilt

Ben starts by addressing his relationship with God. He sets his alarm thirty minutes earlier. Instead of reaching for his phone, he sits in silence for five minutes. He just breathes and prays honestly, "God, I'm exhausted. I feel nothing. I don't know what I'm doing. Help me." There is no performance or pretense, just raw honesty.

He starts reading Scripture again, not out of duty but hunger. He finds Psalms speaking to his weariness. He lingers on verses instead of skimming. Slowly, prayer stops feeling like shouting into a void and starts feeling like a conversation.

He talks to Sarah—really talks to her. He is not deflecting, defending, or minimizing. "I've been drowning. I didn't want to admit it. I'm sorry I've been distant. I need to change some things."

Sarah doesn't fix him, but she walks with him. They pray together for the first time in months. It's awkward at first, but it's real.

Ben starts sleeping seven hours a night. He resumes training three times a week. His mind clears, his body strengthens, and his heart stabilizes because he's processing emotions instead of suppressing them. Ben's soul reconnects because he's spending time with God daily instead of sporadically.

The center begins to hold.

Ben's Horizontal Rebuilt

Ben reaches out to his old college friend, Matt. They schedule a video call every other week. The first call is awkward. They catch up on surface stuff: jobs, kids, sports. But by the third call, Ben admits he's been struggling. Matt shares that he went through something similar two years ago. They start praying for each other at the end of each call. It's not covenant-level yet, but it's moving toward real connection.

Ben joins a men's group at church. Six guys meet weekly for breakfast before work. They read Scripture, share struggles, hold each other accountable. Ben resists at first. Vulnerability feels dangerous. But after a month, he admits he's been drowning. Two of the guys have been there. They listen. They don't fix him, but they stand with him.

Over time, two of those guys become covenant-level friends. They know what's actually going on in Ben's life. He can call them when things get hard. They check in before he even asks.

They speak truth when he's lying to himself. The horizontal line starts to fill in.

Ben's Vertical Rebuilt

Ben asks one of the older men in the group, Robert, to mentor him. They have coffee once a month. Robert has been married thirty years, raised three kids, and walked through his own dark seasons. He doesn't have all the answers, but he has perspective. He asks Ben hard questions and calls out patterns Ben can't see. Robert reminds Ben of truths Ben has forgotten.

Robert challenges Ben's overwork. "You're running yourself into the ground. Why?"

Ben deflects at first. "I'm providing for my family."

Robert pushes. "Are you providing, or are you hiding?"

Ben realizes he's been using work to avoid facing his own emptiness.

Robert doesn't let him off the hook, but he doesn't condemn him either. He walks with him through it.

The vertical line above starts to form.

Ben also starts investing below. One of the younger guys at work, Daniel, is sharp but directionless. Ben invites him to lunch. He shares what he's learning about stewardship, prioritizing family, and not sacrificing one's soul for career advancement.

Daniel starts asking questions.

They meet every couple weeks.

Ben doesn't have all the answers, but he's intentional about sharing what he's walked through.

Ben also starts discipling his sons more intentionally. He is not just managing their behavior but forming their character. He takes his older son on walks and talks about what it means to be a man who follows God. He prays with both boys at bedtime, not rushed prayers but real conversations with God that his sons hear.

The vertical line below begins to take shape.

The Result: A Cross That Bears Weight

Ben's relational cross is no longer empty. The center holds because he's stewarding his relationship with God, his marriage, and his own heart, mind, body, and soul. The horizontal line supports him through covenant friendships that share burdens and speak truth. The vertical line above provides wisdom and perspective. The vertical line below gives him purpose beyond himself.

When work gets stressful now, Ben has people to process with. When his marriage hits friction, he talks to Robert and gets perspective. When his soul feels dry, his men's group prays with him and reminds him he's not alone. When he's tempted to quit training, his accountability partner texts him: "You coming tomorrow morning?"

The cross is bearing weight because the structure is in place. Ben isn't isolated anymore. He's connected. And that connection is saving his life.

PRACTICE PROMPT—PART 3

❖ Draw your relational cross again. This time, fill in names at every level:

- **Center**: You + God (+ spouse if married)
- **Horizontal, Covenant level:** 1–3 people
- **Horizontal, Middle circle:** 5–10 people
- **Horizontal, Outer circle:** List a few key acquaintances
- **Vertical, Above:** 1–2 mentors
- **Vertical, Below:** 1–3 people you're investing in

❖ Commit to one action per axis this month:

- **Center:** One daily practice to steward your relationship with God and yourself (and spouse if married)
- **Horizontal:** Reach out to one covenant or middle-circle friend weekly
- **Vertical, Above:** Schedule one conversation with a mentor
- **Vertical, Below:** Invest intentionally in one person below you

Success Criteria

☐ You drew your cross with actual names (not just categories).

☐ You executed all four commitments for at least three out of four weeks.

 ☐ You can identify one specific way each axis strengthened you this month.

Troubleshooting

If your cross is still mostly empty after this exercise, you're either not engaging with people around you, or you're waiting for relationships to magically appear. Relationships require initiative. Reach out and invite people to join you.

If you completed the actions but felt no difference, you might be going through the motions without genuine engagement. Relationships require presence and not just attendance.

If you struggled with the vertical above (mentorship), your pride is blocking you. Humble yourself and ask for help.

If you struggled with vertical below (investment), you're underestimating what you have to offer. Someone needs what you've learned.

FINAL WARNINGS

Most people don't lose their relational cross in one dramatic explosion. It erodes slowly. These are the patterns that kill connection before you realize it's dying.

Warning 1: Confusing Busy with Connected

You attend church, you work with colleagues, and you see neighbors. Your calendar is full, but when life gets hard, you have no one to call. Proximity doesn't equal connection. Activity doesn't equal relationship. If you can't name two people who know what's actually going on inside you, you're isolated even if you're never alone.

The fix is to stop saying yes to every invitation and start investing deeply in two or three people. Cancel the coffee date with an acquaintance to have dinner with a covenant friend. Quality beats quantity every time.

Warning 2: Sacrificing the Center to Build the Cross

You pour into everyone else while your own heart, mind, body, and soul deteriorate. You tell yourself it's service. It's not. It's depletion masquerading as generosity. Eventually, you have nothing left to give, and the relationships you sacrificed yourself for collapse under the weight of your burnout.

Jesus withdrew to pray, as mentioned in Luke 5:16. He protected the center so he could sustain the work. If Jesus needed time alone with the Father, you definitely do. Steward yourself first. It's not selfish. It's prerequisite.

Warning 3: Letting Toxic People Stay Too Long

Proverbs 13:20 warns that the companion of fools will suffer harm. Some people are draining. Some relationships are toxic. You keep giving them access to the inner circle because you feel guilty about setting boundaries, or you think they need you, or you're afraid of being judgmental. Meanwhile, they're corroding your peace, your clarity, and your capacity to serve others well.

Healthy boundaries aren't rejection. They're wisdom. Move toxic people to the outer circle or off the cross entirely. Protect what God is building in you.

Warning 4: Pride Blocking Mentorship

You tell yourself you don't need a mentor. You've figured it out. You're self-sufficient. But your marriage is strained and you don't know how to fix it. Your career has plateaued and you're stuck. Your spiritual life feels dry and you don't know how to reconnect. These are exactly the areas where someone ten years ahead could help, but pride keeps you from asking.

Proverbs 12:15 says the way of a fool is right in his own eyes, but a wise man listens to advice. Humble yourself. Find someone who has walked where you're walking. Ask for help.

Warning 5: Isolation Hardening Into Identity

You've been alone so long you've stopped noticing. You tell yourself you're introverted, you don't need people, and you're fine. But you're not fine. Your heart is unstable because no one corrects your thinking. Because no one challenges your assumptions, your mind is narrow. Your soul is dry because you're trying to follow God in isolation, which he never designed you to do.

Hebrews 10:24–25 commands not neglecting to meet together.

If your cross is empty and you're reading this, you're in danger. Reach out this week. Join a group. Ask someone to coffee. Build the cross before the isolation kills you.

Warning 6: Using Relationships to Avoid God
Another danger is when relationships become your entire source of meaning, comfort, and identity. You need constant affirmation and can't handle being alone. You make friends into saviors. When they inevitably fail you, you're crushed.

Relationships support the soul. They don't replace communion with God. Your spouse isn't your savior and your mentor isn't infallible. Your friends can't fix what only God can heal. Build the horizontal and vertical, but anchor everything at the center in your relationship with God.

The Pattern
These warnings all point to the same root issue: misplaced weight. Either you're carrying too much alone (isolation), giving too much to the wrong people (toxic relationships), or expecting people to carry what only God can (idolatry). The relational cross works when the center is anchored in God, when boundaries protect what he's building, and when you invest wisely in the horizontal and vertical.

STEWARDING THE CROSS

Believe it or not, relationships are not optional for wellness. Scripture commands connection, and science confirms necessity. Your relational cross determines how long you last, how well you serve, and how deeply you love.

The center must hold. Steward your relationship with God. If you're married, steward your covenant with your spouse. Take care of your own heart, mind, body, and soul. You cannot give what you do not have. Fill the center first.

Build the horizontal. Covenant friendships should be where burdens are shared and truth is spoken. Middle-circle relationships are where community and encouragement flow. Outer-circle connections provide breadth and opportunity. Don't try to make everyone covenant level. Steward intensity with wisdom.

Engage the vertical. Seek mentors who have walked where you're walking. Receive their wisdom with humility. Pour into those coming behind you, and give away what you've been given. Generativity is not optional for mature faith.

Relationships amplify The SCAL Method. A sound heart steadies your relational presence. A sound mind sharpens relational discernment. A strong body extends relational capacity. A strong soul anchors relational purpose. Train the four arenas, and your relationships strengthen. Neglect them, and your relationships suffer.

The relational cross is not a program. It's a framework for stewardship. Take up your cross daily. Stand at the center. Invest deeply in the horizontal. Discern carefully above, and give generously below. Steward the cross wisely.

"A cord of three strands is not quickly broken" (Ecclesiastes 4:12).

You are one strand, God is another, and relationships are the third. Woven together, they create strength that isolation cannot provide.

Build the cross. Steward the cross. Let it bear the weight of your life so you can bear the weight of service without collapsing.

CONCLUSION

WHAT YOU'VE GAINED

You now have something many people don't: a way to actually live out the Great Commandment. Don't just know it, but live it. Love God with all your heart. You've got the framework. Name what you're feeling, and accept it without suppression. Analyze where it's coming from, and express it without destruction. Reframe distortions before they harden into bitterness. That's not therapy. That's discipleship. Train the heart and the ripple effect is real.

Love God with all your mind. You know how this works now. Perceive what's actually happening instead of what you think is happening. Comprehend the meaning accurately. Evaluate with evidence, not emotion. Decide based on truth, and act with conviction. A sound mind protects you from your own reactivity and from everyone trying to manipulate you. Wisdom isn't inherited. It's cultivated. You have the tools.

Love God with all your strength. The body is a temple requiring maintenance. You train, recover, adapt, repeat. It's not for vanity but for longevity. Physical discipline extends your ministry runway. It stabilizes your emotions and sharpens your thinking. A strong body creates capacity to serve for decades instead of burning out within years.

Love God with all your soul. Pray, read Scripture, worship, and fast. These aren't optional add-ons. They're the foundation. You receive from God. You reflect on what He's saying and respond in obedience. Repeat daily. When the soul is nourished, resilience flows into every other arena. When it's dry, everything else becomes brittle.

The endurance chapter taught you how to sustain these disciplines under pressure and how to stay under the load when everything in you wants to quit. Strategic discomfort builds capacity across all four arenas.

The relationships chapter showed you where the four arenas get tested. It also taught you about the relational cross: who belongs where, how close, and how much weight they carry. Connection heals what isolation corrodes.

Most importantly, the four arenas work together. They're not separate compartments. A sound heart steadies the mind. A sound mind trains the heart. A strong body stabilizes both. A strong soul anchors everything. What happens in one arena ripples into the others. Always.

Now comes the work.

THE PEOPLE YOU'VE MET

Throughout this book, you met people who started where you are now.

Sarah is the worship leader whose unchecked anger nearly destroyed her Sunday morning ministry. She learned to name, accept, analyze, express, and reframe her emotions. Training her heart changed how she led, how she spoke, and how she carried herself in public.

Jade received critical feedback at work. She had two options: react defensively and escalate the conflict, or pause, perceive accurately, evaluate rationally, and respond professionally. She chose the second path. A sound mind protected her from her own reactivity.

Craig had a desk job. He was thirty-five. He faced two futures: neglect his body and burn out by forty-five, or steward his temple and serve faithfully for decades. The body determines how long you can show up. Craig chose longevity.

Desmond is the worship pastor whose soul was starving. Prayer felt dutiful. Scripture felt dead. He committed to receiving from God daily, reflecting on what he heard, responding in obedience, and repeating the cycle. By month three, his wife noticed the shift. By year one, his ministry was stronger than it had been in years. A strong soul creates a legacy.

Alicia could start strong but couldn't sustain. She lacked endurance. When things got hard, she quit. Strategic discomfort changed that. She learned to remain under the load. Her body strengthened and emotions steadied. Alicia's spiritual life deepened, and her endurance built her capacity across all four arenas.

Ben was drowning in isolation while surrounded by people. His relational cross was out of balance. He rebuilt it: reciprocal friendships on the horizontal, mentors above him and investment below him on the vertical. Connection healed what isolation had corroded.

These people are not perfect. They are faithful. All of them are steadier. All of them have capacity they didn't have before.

That can be your story, too.

WHEN YOU FAIL

You will fail. It's not a question of if but when.

You'll skip a week, or let emotions run unchecked. You'll coast mentally, neglect your body, or let prayer slide. It happens. We're human.

What matters is what you do after you fail.

Failure is data. It shows you where you need help, where your systems are weak, and where pride convinced you that you could coast.

When you fail, do this:

- Confess it.
- Identify the breakdown.
- Adjust the system.
- Start again immediately.

Confess it. Name the failure without excuse. "I stopped showing up. I let my heart run wild. I neglected prayer." No spin. Just truth.

Identify the breakdown. Was it lack of accountability? Was it overcommitment, pride, or chaos? Figure out what broke and why.

Adjust the system. If you missed a week because you had no accountability, text someone and ask them to check in. If you skipped prayer because mornings are chaos, move it to lunch. Don't just restart. Recalibrate.

Start again immediately. Don't wait until Monday or next month. Do it Today. Make one micro move in each arena. Name one emotion. Read one verse. Do ten pushups. Pray for three minutes. Then do it again tomorrow.

The difference between a setback and a surrender is what you do next. Setbacks are normal. Surrender is the only true failure.

"If we confess our sins, he is faithful and just to forgive us our sins and to cleanse us from all unrighteousness" (First John 1:9).

Grace doesn't excuse laziness, but it does cover failure. Confess. Adjust. Restart. The work continues.

THE 30/90/365 DAY VISION

Progress isn't linear. But patterns emerge. Here's what the next year looks like if you stay faithful.

The First Thirty Days: Establishing Rhythm

The first month is not about results. It's about building the habit of showing up. Expect resistance and awkwardness. Expect to forget some days and scramble to catch up.

Focus on the basics:

- **Heart:** Practice naming and reframing one emotion daily.
- **Mind:** Walk through the decision process with one choice per day.
- **Body:** Train three times per week, even if just twenty minutes.
- **Soul:** Commit to ten minutes of Scripture and prayer daily.

Track it. Use a notebook, a spreadsheet, or an app.

Accountability matters. At the end of thirty days, you'll have data. You'll see patterns and know where you need help.

Months two to three: Pushing Through Resistance

This is the danger zone. The novelty has worn off. Progress feels slow. You'll be tempted to quit. Don't.

Months two and three are where you build grit. This is where most people abandon the work, convinced it's not working. But it is working. You're just in the unseen-growth phase. Roots go deep before fruit appears. You'll notice the following:

- Your emotional reactivity is decreasing. You catch yourself before snapping.
- Your thinking is sharper. You ask better questions. You spot manipulation faster.
- Your body feels steadier. You're sleeping better. You have more capacity.
- Your soul feels less brittle. Prayer doesn't feel dutiful. Scripture speaks.

These are small shifts. But they compound. Push through.

Year 1: Visible Transformation

By month twelve, the changes are undeniable. Others notice. You notice. The four arenas aren't mastered. They never will be. But they're trained.

Here's what you'll see after one year:

Your heart is steadier, and you don't spiral into resentment or anxiety as quickly. You name emotions before they control you. Words you speak carry life instead of corrosion.

Your mind is sharper. You think critically. You weigh evidence and question assumptions. Your discernment holds under pressure. Fallacies are easier for you to recognize, and you resist manipulation.

Your body is stronger. You have capacity you didn't have before. You can serve longer, love steadier, endure harder circumstances without breaking. Recovery happens faster, and your resilience is deeper.

Your soul is anchored because prayer is rhythmic, Scripture is nourishing, and worship is honest. Community is life-giving. You can sit in spiritual dryness without abandoning the disciplines.

This isn't perfection. This is formation. You're no longer the same person who started.

BEYOND YEAR 1

This isn't a twelve-week program. This is a lifelong practice. Year one builds the foundation. Year two deepens the capacity. By year five, the disciplines are automatic. By year ten, you're teaching them to the next generation.

The work never ends. It does get easier, and the fruit multiplies.

THE RIPPLE EFFECT

What you do with your heart, mind, body, and soul doesn't stay with you. It ripples outward.

Your marriage changes because you're changing. When you train your heart, your spouse feels it. You stop reacting and start responding. Before resentment can calcify, you name it. You accept grief without projecting it onto your partner. Words you speak are steadier, and your presence becomes safe. Emotional regulation becomes relational transformation.

Your children are watching everything. They see you think critically, question assumptions, and weigh evidence. They learn discernment by watching you model it. Your intellectual integrity becomes their inheritance. Your children watch you choose the hard thing when comfort calls and learn that stewarding the temple matters. They hear you pray. They see Scripture open on the table and notice when you withdraw to be with God. Observing you teaches them that communion with God isn't optional.

How long can you serve? A strong body answers that question. You don't burn out at forty-five. You serve faithfully into your sixties, seventies, and eighties. Physical discipline isn't vanity. It's longevity for the sake of service. A sound heart makes you safe for people in crisis.

People come to you because they know you won't react in anger, judge in disgust, or collapse under their pain. A sound mind makes you trustworthy in leadership.

People follow you because your thinking is clear, decisions are sound, and discernment is sharp. A strong soul makes you resilient in trial. When the storm comes, and it will, you don't abandon God. You remain faithful. You model endurance.

The people around you absorb what you live. Your home becomes a place where emotions are named, not suppressed. Your workplace becomes a place where critical thinking is modeled, not assumed. Your church becomes a place where spiritual disciplines are practiced, not just preached.

Legacy isn't only financial. It's the patterns you pass down. Model this. Live this. Make it ordinary.

THE THEOLOGICAL FOUNDATION

Mark 12:30–31 isn't just the organizing verse for this book. It's the organizing command for your life:

"Love the Lord your God with all your heart and with all your soul and with all your mind and with all your strength. The second is this: Love your neighbor as yourself" (Mark 12:30–31).

The SCAL Method doesn't add to this command. It gives you equipment to fulfill it. Heart, Mind, Body, and Soul are the four arenas for one integrated life. We have one purpose: to love God with everything and overflow that love to others.

Training your heart isn't self-help. It's stewarding the control center of your emotions so resentment doesn't poison your witness and anger doesn't destroy your relationships.

Sharpening your mind isn't intellectualism. It's cultivating the discernment needed to distinguish truth from lies and resist the manipulation of a fallen world.

Strengthening your body isn't vanity. It's stewarding the temple so you can serve faithfully for decades instead of burning out within years.

Nourishing your soul isn't religious performance. It's communion with the God who made you, sustains you, and calls you to love him with everything you are.

Endurance sustains this love under pressure. Relationships express this love in community.

This is stewardship. This is discipleship. This is faithfulness.

WHAT THIS BOOK IS NOT

This book isn't therapy. It's not pastoral counseling. It's not a guarantee that you'll never struggle again.

If you're in crisis, get professional help. When you're spiritually dry, talk to your pastor. If you're battling clinical depression, see a counselor. The SCAL Method complements those supports. It doesn't replace them.

This is a framework for stewardship. It's a blueprint for whole-person discipleship. It's a map for faithfulness over the long haul.

Use it well.

WHERE I AM NOW

I'm still working this out. My relational cross is still thin. Some mornings, prayer feels dry. I still catch myself letting emotions drive me instead of regulating them. I'm not where I was three years ago, but I'm not where I want to be, either.

The frameworks work, not because they're perfect but because they allow me to be faithful. I show up. I do the work, fail, and restart. The progress is real even when it's slow.

That's what I want you to hear: you don't have to have it all figured out. You just have to start. Make one micro move. Get through one day, then another. The discipline builds. The capacity grows. The fruit comes.

I coach people for a living. Even though I pour into others constantly, I still need people pouring into me. I still need accountability and someone to call me out when I'm lying to myself. Being sound enough to keep my emotions in check, and to remain free from manipulation is still something I need. I still need to be physically strong and have encounters with God. The work never ends. I don't want it to, either.

BEGINNING TODAY

The practice prompts scattered throughout this book aren't one-time exercises. Return to them quarterly. Cycle through them as your capacity deepens. The prompts grow with you.

Start small. Pick one arena that's weakest right now, and commit to one discipline this week. Just one.

Does your heart feel brittle? Name and reframe one emotion daily for seven days.

Is your mind feeling foggy? Walk through one decision this week with full attention to the process.

Does your body feel neglected? Train three times this week, even if it's just fifteen minutes.

Is your soul feeling dry? Spend ten minutes in Scripture and five minutes in prayer daily.

Notice what changes. The work isn't complicated. It's consistent.

"Above all else, guard your heart, for everything you do flows from it" (Proverbs 4:23).

Guarding your heart isn't passive protection. It's active stewardship. The same applies to your mind, your body, and your soul. Guard them. Train them. Steward them.

THE FINAL WORD

"Love the Lord your God with all your heart and with all your soul and with all your mind and with all your strength" (Mark 12:30).

This is the command. This is the blueprint. This is the call.

Train your heart so your words carry life instead of corrosion. Sharpen your mind so your discernment holds under pressure. Strengthen your body so you can serve longer and love steadier. Nourish your soul so resilience flows into everything else.

This is stewardship. This is discipleship. This is faithfulness.

God gives strength for what He commands. Show up. Do the work. Trust the process.

The fruit will come: patience, steadiness, and love that lasts.

You will live a life worthy of the calling. Begin today. Keep going tomorrow.

Finish the race.

FINAL PRACTICE PROMPT

- ❖ Write down your plan for the next thirty days:
  - **Heart:** Name one emotional pattern you will reframe daily using the framework.
  - **Mind:** Name one area where you will practice critical evaluation this week.
  - **Body:** Choose one physical practice to do three times per week.
  - **Soul:** Choose one spiritual rhythm you will defend daily.Text this plan to one person who will check in with you weekly. Accountability is not optional.

Success Criteria

☐ You wrote specific commitments for all four arenas (not vague intentions like "Be better").

☐ You texted your commitments to someone within twenty-four hours.

☐ That person agreed to check in weekly, and you responded when they checked in the first time.

Troubleshooting

If you couldn't identify specific practices, go back and review one chapter summary. Pick the simplest item from each arena to start.

If you wrote vague commitments, make them measurable: instead of "Pray more," write "Pray for ten minutes every morning before coffee."

If you haven't texted anyone yet, you might be overthinking whom to ask. Pick someone who cares about you and send it now—imperfect accountability beats no accountability.

If the person you texted hasn't checked in after a week, they might have forgotten or not understood you were serious. Follow up: "Hey, can you text me this Sunday to ask about my thirty-day plan?"

If you feel overwhelmed by committing to all four arenas, start with two (pick your weakest areas), and add the others after thirty days.

VERSE LIST

Introduction—The Foundation

- "Love the Lord your God with all your heart and with all your soul and with all your mind and with all your strength. The second is this: 'Love your neighbor as yourself'" (Mark 12:30–31).
- "A sound heart is life to the body, but envy is rottenness to the bones" (Proverbs 14:30).
- "The Lord gives wisdom; from his mouth come knowledge and understanding" (Proverbs 2:6).
- "Your bodies are temples of the Holy Spirit... honor God with your bodies" (1 Corinthians 6:19–20).
- "He restores my soul" (Psalm 23:3).

Introduction—Arena Interconnection

- "Be transformed by the renewal of your mind" (Romans 12:2).

Introduction—Framework as Discipleship

- "Above all else, guard your heart, for everything you do flows from it" (Proverbs 4:23).

Introduction—Stewardship =/=Perfection

- Matthew 25:14–30 gives us The Parable of the Talents.

Introduction—The Road Ahead

- Mark 12:30–31 is repeated for emphasis.

A Sound Heart

- "A sound heart is life to the body, but envy is rottenness to the bones" (Proverbs 14:30).
- "Above all else, guard your heart, for everything you do flows from it" (Proverbs 4:23).

A Sound Heart—Exegesis

- Proverbs 14:30 is repeated for exegesis.
- "For you shall worship no other god, for the Lord, whose name is Jealous, is a jealous God" (Exodus 34:14).
- "Let us not become conceited, provoking one another, envying one another" (Galatians 5:26).

A Sound Heart—Physical Consequence

- "When I kept silent, my bones wasted away . . . my strength was sapped as in the heat of summer" (Psalm 32:3–4).

A Sound Heart—Groundwork and Sequence

- Proverbs 4:23 (Name)
- Psalm 42 (Accept)
- Proverbs 14:30 (Analyze)
- Ephesians 4:26 (Express)
- Romans 12:2 (Reframe)

A Sound Heart—Reframing Discipline

- Romans 12:2 is repeated for emphasis.

A Sound Heart—Common Reframing Pitfalls

- Grief must be faced not bypassed. "Jesus wept" (John 11:35).
- Isaiah 30:10 gives us a warning against false peace.

A Sound Heart—Practice Schedule

- "I have stored up your word in my heart, that I might not sin against you" (Psalm 119:11).

A Sound Heart—A Level Deeper

- "A man without self-control is like a city broken into and left without walls" (Proverbs 25:28).

A Sound Heart—Integrating

- "Do not be anxious about anything . . . the peace of God will guard your hearts" (Philippians 4:6–7).
- "Confess your sins to one another and pray for one another, that you may be healed" (James 5:16).
- "I am fearfully and wonderfully made" (Psalm 139:14).
- "I will never leave you nor forsake you" (Hebrews 13:5).
- Ephesians 6:17 shows that Scripture is the sword of the Spirit.

A Sound Heart—Markers of Progress

- "The fruit of the Spirit is love, joy, peace, patience, kindness, goodness, faithfulness, gentleness, self-control" (Galatians 5:22–23).

A Sound Heart—Final Notes and Warnings

- "I discipline my body and keep it under control" (1 Corinthians 9:27).

A Sound Heart—Conclusion

- I can do all things through him who strengthens me" (Philippians 4:13).

A Sound Mind—Understanding a Sound Mind

- "For God hath not given us the spirit of fear; but of power, and of love, and of a sound mind" (2 Timothy 1:7).

A Sound Mind—Verse, Context, and Word

- 2 Timothy 1:7 is repeated for exegesis.

A Sound Mind—Wisdom Types and Sources

- "For where envying and strife is, there is confusion and every evil work. But the wisdom that is from above is first pure, then peaceable, gentle, and easy to be intreated, full of mercy and good fruits, without partiality, and without hypocrisy. And the fruit of righteousness is sown in peace of them that make peace" (James 3:16–18).
- "If any of you lack wisdom, let him ask of God, that giveth to all men liberally, and upbraideth not; and it shall be given him" (James 1:5).
- "The fear of the Lord is the beginning of wisdom: and the knowledge of the holy is understanding" (Proverbs 9:10).
- "For wisdom is better than rubies; and all the things that may be desired are not to be compared to it" (Proverbs 8:11).
- "How much better is it to get wisdom than gold! and to get understanding rather to be chosen than silver" (Proverbs 16:16).

A Sound Mind—Examining Sacred Beliefs

- "Taste and see that the Lord is good" (Psalm 34:8).
- "Test everything; hold fast what is good" (1 Thessalonians 5:21).

A Sound Mind—How Meditation Helps

- "So then faith cometh by hearing, and hearing by the word of God" (Romans 10:17).
- "Now faith is the substance of things hoped for, the evidence of things not seen" (Hebrews 11:1).

- "But his delight is in the law of the Lord; and in his law doth he meditate day and night" (Psalm 1:2).

A Sound Mind—Others' Faulty Arguments
- "The simple believes everything, but the prudent gives thought to his steps" (Proverbs 14:15).
- "The one who states his case first seems right, until the other comes and examines him" (Proverbs 18:17).
- Galatians 1:8 says that even angels can preach falsely.
- Acts 17:11 says that the Bereans examined the Scriptures daily.
- "If one gives an answer before he hears, it is his folly and shame" (Proverbs 18:13).
- "Be quick to hear, slow to speak, slow to anger" (James 1:19).
- Matthew 7:13–14 says few find the narrow path.
- "There is a way that seems right to a man, but its end is the way to death" (Proverbs 14:12).

A Strong and Healthy Body
- 1 Corinthians 6:19–20—"Your body is the temple of the Holy Spirit... Therefore glorify God in your body and in your spirit which are God's."
- Proverbs 27:17—"As iron sharpens iron, so one person sharpens another."

A Strong and Healthy Body—Temple Stewardship
- 1 Corinthians 6:19–20 (repeated for emphasis)
- Psalm 139:14—"I am fearfully and wonderfully made."

A Strong and Healthy Body—Strategic Metabolic Stress
- Matthew 6:16–18—Jesus on proper motive for fasting
- Isaiah 58—God's chosen fast: justice and mercy
- Psalm 63:1—"My soul thirsts for you; my flesh faints for you."

A Strong and Healthy Body—Final Warnings: Guardrails
- 1 Corinthians 9:27—"I discipline my body and keep it under control."
- Romans 12:1—"Present your bodies as a living sacrifice."

A Strong and Healthy Soul
- Psalm 1:2–3—Like a tree planted by streams of water
- 2 Timothy 1:7—God gave us a spirit of power, love, and self—

control (sōphronismos)

A Strong and Healthy Soul—Biblical Foundation
- Genesis 2:7—God breathed life into man
- Psalm 139:13—15—Fearfully and wonderfully made
- Jeremiah 1:5—Before I formed you in the womb
- 2 Timothy 3:16—17—All Scripture is breathed out by God
- Psalm 23:2—3—He leads me beside still waters

A Strong and Healthy Soul—Practice 1: Scripture Intake
- 2 Timothy 3:16—17—All Scripture is breathed out by God

A Strong and Healthy Soul—Practice 2: Prayer
- 1 Thessalonians 5:17—Pray without ceasing

A Strong and Healthy Soul—Practice 3: Worship
- Hebrews 10:24—25—Do not neglect meeting together

A Strong and Healthy Soul—Practice 4: Fasting
- Matthew 6:16—When you fast

A Strong and Healthy Soul—Cultivating Character
- Galatians 5:22—23—The fruit of the Spirit

A Strong and Healthy Soul—Spiritual Warfare
- Ephesians 6:12—We wrestle against spiritual forces
- Ephesians 6:13—17—The armor of God

A Strong and Healthy Soul—When Things Get Silent
- Job 13:15—Though he slay me, I will hope in him
- Psalm 13:1—2—How long, O Lord?
- Matthew 27:46—My God, my God, why have you forsaken me?
- Hebrews 13:8—The same yesterday, today, and forever

A Strong and Healthy Soul—Spiritual Community
- Proverbs 27:17—Iron sharpens iron
- Hebrews 10:24—25—Do not neglect meeting together

A Strong and Healthy Soul—SCAL Method Integration
- 3 John 1:2—In good health, as it goes well with your soul
- Proverbs 4:22—God's words are healing to all flesh
- Psalm 103:3—Who heals all your diseases

A Strong and Healthy Soul—Measuring Spiritual Progress
- Galatians 5:22—23—The fruit of the Spirit

Endurance and Strategic Discomfort
- Romans 5:3–4—"And not only so, but we glory in tribulations also: knowing that tribulation worketh patience; and patience, experience; and experience, hope."
- Hebrews 12:1—"Wherefore seeing we also are compassed about with so great a cloud of witnesses, let us lay aside every weight, and the sin which doth so easily beset us, and let us run with patience the race that is set before us."

Endurance and Strategic Discomfort—The Call To Endure
- James 1:2–3—"My brethren, count it all joy when ye fall into divers temptations; knowing this, that the trying of your faith worketh patience."
- James 4:7—"Submit yourselves therefore to God. Resist the devil, and he will flee from you."
- Romans 12:12—"Rejoicing in hope; patient in tribulation; continuing instant in prayer."
- Romans 5:3–5 (repeated for exegesis)
- Deuteronomy 8:2—God led Israel through the wilderness to test them
- Deuteronomy 1:2—The journey that should have taken 11 days took 40 years

Endurance and Strategic Discomfort—Spiritual Endurance
- James 1:12—"Blessed is the man that endureth temptation: for when he is tried, he shall receive the crown of life, which the Lord hath promised to them that love him."
- Revelation 2:10—"Be thou faithful unto death, and I will give thee a crown of life."
- Hebrews 11:13–16—The heroes of faith looking forward to the heavenly city
- Hebrews 11:24–26—Moses choosing reproach over Egypt's treasures

Endurance and Strategic Discomfort—Four Critical Mistakes
- 1 Corinthians 9:27—"But I keep under my body, and bring it into subjection: lest that by any means, when I have preached

to others, I myself should be a castaway."
- Philippians 2:3–4—Esteem others better than yourself; look to others' interests

Endurance and Strategic Discomfort—The Invitation
- Philippians 4:13—"I can do all things through Christ which strengtheneth me."

The Relational Cross—A House of Wellness
- Luke 9:23—"If anyone would come after me, let him deny himself and take up his cross daily and follow me."
- Acts 2:42—Koinonia (fellowship/partnership)
- Ruth 1:16—Hesed (covenant love)
- Matthew 17:1—Jesus with Peter, James, John at the Transfiguration
- Matthew 26:37—Jesus takes Peter, James, John to Gethsemane
- Mark 5:37—Jesus takes three to raising of Jairus' daughter
- Luke 10:1—The seventy-two sent out
- Luke 5:16—Jesus withdrew to pray
- Mark 1:35—Jesus withdrew early morning to pray
- Luke 6:12—Jesus prayed all night
- Matthew 4:1—Jesus in the wilderness
- Proverbs 17:17—"A friend loves at all times"
- Proverbs 27:17—"Iron sharpens iron"

The Relational Cross—The Center Point
- Mark 12:31—"Love your neighbor as yourself"
- Genesis 2:24—Covenant of marriage: two become one flesh
- Ephesians 5:28–29—Husbands love wives as their own bodies
- 1 Corinthians 12—The body as interconnected parts

The Relational Cross—The Horizontal Axis
- 1 Samuel 18:1—Jonathan's soul knit to David's soul
- 1 Samuel 20—Jonathan protects David
- Galatians 6:10—"Do good to everyone, especially household of faith"
- Galatians 6:2—"Bear one another's burdens"
- Proverbs 18:24—A friend who sticks closer than a brother
- Proverbs 27:9—The sweetness of earnest counsel
- Proverbs 12:15—"A wise man listens to advice"

The Relational Cross—The Vertical Axis
- Hebrews 13:7—"Remember your leaders"
- 2 Timothy 2:2—"Entrust to faithful men"
- Proverbs 13:20—"Whoever walks with the wise becomes wise"
- 1 Corinthians 3:5–7—Paul and Apollos as servants

The Relational Cross—Intensity and Distance
- Proverbs 25:17—"Let your foot be seldom in your neighbor's house"
- 1 Corinthians 15:33—"Bad company corrupts good morals"

The Relational Cross—How Relationships Integrate
- Hebrews 10:24–25—"Stir up one another to love and good works"

The Relational Cross—Conclusion
- Ecclesiastes 4:12—"A cord of three strands is not quickly broken"

Conclusion—When You Fail
- 1 John 1:9—"If we confess our sins, he is faithful and just to forgive us our sins and to cleanse us from all unrighteousness."

Conclusion—Begin Today
- Proverbs 4:23—"Above all else, guard your heart, for everything you do flows from it."

Conclusion—The Final Word
- Mark 12:30—"Love the Lord your God with all your heart and with all your soul and with all your mind and with all your strength."

SOURCES

Introduction—The Foundation

Wright, N. T. *Paul and the Faithfulness of God*. Minneapolis: Fortress Press, 2013.

Willard, Dallas. *Renovation of the Heart*. Colorado Springs, CO: NavPress, 2002.

Introduction—How the Four Arenas Interconnect

Gross, James J. "Emotion Regulation: Conceptual and Empirical Foundations." In *Handbook of Emotion Regulation*, edited by James J. Gross, 3–20. New York: Guilford Press, 2014.

Sapolsky, Robert M. *Why Zebras Don't Get Ulcers*. New York: Holt, 2004.

Introduction—The SCAL Framework as Discipleship

Foster, Richard J. *Celebration of Discipline*. San Francisco: HarperSanFrancisco, 1998.

Peterson, Eugene H. *Christ Plays in Ten Thousand Places*. Grand Rapids, MI: Eerdmans, 2005.

Introduction—Stewardship, Not Perfection

Cloud, Henry, and John Townsend. *Boundaries*. Grand Rapids, MI: Zondervan, 1992.

Seligman, Martin E. P. *Flourish*. New York: Free Press, 2011.

A Sound Heart—Understanding a Sound Heart

Brown, Francis, S. R. Driver, and Charles A. Briggs. *A Hebrew and English Lexicon of the Old Testament*. Oxford: Clarendon Press, 1906.

A Sound Heart—Biblical Foundation and Exegesis

Waltke, Bruce K. *The Book of Proverbs: Chapters 15–31*. Grand Rapids, MI: Eerdmans, 2005.

Wright, N. T. *Paul and the Faithfulness of God*. Minneapolis: Fortress Press, 2013.

A Sound Heart—Emotions and Physical Consequence

McEwen, Bruce S. "Protective and Damaging Effects of Stress Mediators." *New England Journal of Medicine* 338, no. 3 (1998): 171–79. https://doi.org/10.1056/NEJM199801153380307.

Sapolsky, Robert M. *Why Zebras Don't Get Ulcers*. New York: Holt, 2004.

A Sound Heart—Training Your Emotions

Lieberman, Matthew D., Tristen K. Inagaki, Golnaz Tabibnia, and

Molly J. Crockett. "Putting Feelings into Words: Affect Labeling Disrupts Amygdala Activity." *Psychological Science* 18, no. 5 (2007): 421–28. https://doi.org/10.1111/j.1467-9280.2007.01916.x.

A Sound Heart—Reframing Discipline

Beck, Aaron T. *Cognitive Therapy and the Emotional Disorders*. New York: Penguin, 1979.

Gross, James J. "Emotion Regulation: Conceptual and Empirical Foundations." In *Handbook of Emotion Regulation*, edited by James J. Gross, 3–20. New York: Guilford Press, 2014.

Ochsner, Kevin N., and James J. Gross. "The Cognitive Control of Emotion." *Trends in Cognitive Sciences* 9, no. 5 (2005): 242–49. https://doi.org/10.1016/j.tics.2005.03.010.

A Sound Heart—Common Reframing Pitfalls

Bonanno, George A. *The Other Side of Sadness*. New York: Basic Books, 2009.

Janoff-Bulman, Ronnie. *Shattered Assumptions*. New York: Free Press, 1992.

A Sound Heart—Practice Schedule for Reframing

Pennebaker, James W. *Opening Up: The Healing Power of Expressing Emotions*. New York: Guilford Press, 1997.

A Sound Heart—Emotional Intelligence

Goleman, Daniel. *Emotional Intelligence*. New York: Bantam Books, 1995.

Gross, James J., and Ross A. Thompson. "Emotion Regulation: Conceptual Foundations." In *Handbook of Emotion Regulation*, edited by James J. Gross, 3–24. New York: Guilford Press, 2007.

Salovey, Peter, and John D. Mayer. "Emotional Intelligence." *Imagination, Cognition and Personality* 9, no. 3 (1990): 185–211. https://doi.org/10.2190/DUGG-P24E-52WK-6CDG.

A Sound Mind—Lexicons

"G4995—sōphronismos." *Blue Letter Bible*. Accessed October 18, 2025. https://www.blueletterbible.org/lexicon/g4995/kjv/tr/0-1/.

"Strong's Greek: 4995. sōphronismos." *BibleHub*. Accessed October 18, 2025. https://biblehub.com/greek/4995.htm.

"Strong's #4995: sōphronismos." *BibleTools*. Accessed October 18, 2025. https://www.bibletools.org/index.cfm/fuseaction/Lexicon.show/ID/G4995/sophronismos.htm.

A Sound Mind—Critical Thinking

Scriven, Michael, and Richard Paul. "Defining Critical Thinking." 8th Annual International Conference on Critical Thinking and Education Reform, 1987. http://www.criticalthinking.org/pages/defining-critical-thinking/766.

University of Louisville. "What Is Critical Thinking?" Accessed October 18, 2025. https://louisville.edu/ideastoaction/about/criticalthinking/what.

University of Hong Kong. "Defining Critical Thinking." Accessed October 18, 2025. https://philosophy.hku.hk/think/critical/definitions.php.

A Sound Mind—Argumentation

Hamblin, C. L. *Fallacies*. London: Methuen, 1970.

Kahneman, Daniel. *Thinking, Fast and Slow*. New York: Farrar, Straus and Giroux, 2011.

Toulmin, Stephen E. *The Uses of Argument*. Updated ed. Cambridge: Cambridge University Press, 2003.

Walton, Douglas N. *Informal Logic: A Pragmatic Approach*. 2nd ed. Cambridge: Cambridge University Press, 2008.

A Strong and Healthy Body—Fasting

de Cabo, Rafael, and Mark P. Mattson. "Effects of Intermittent Fasting on Health, Aging, and Disease." *New England Journal of Medicine* 381, no. 26 (2019): 2541–51.

Longo, Valter D., and Mark P. Mattson. "Fasting: Molecular Mechanisms and Clinical Applications." *Cell Metabolism* 19, no. 2 (2014): 181–92.

A Strong and Healthy Soul—Foundations

Longman, Tremper. *Genesis*. Grand Rapids, MI: Zondervan, 2012.

Waltke, Bruce K. *The Book of Proverbs*. Grand Rapids, MI: Eerdmans, 2004.

A Strong and Healthy Soul—Spiritual Formation

Foster, Richard J. *Prayer: Finding the Heart's True Home*. San Francisco: HarperSanFrancisco, 1992.

Willard, Dallas. *Renovation of the Heart*. Colorado Springs, CO: NavPress, 2002.

Endurance and Strategic Discomfort

Baumeister, Roy F., and John Tierney. *Willpower*. New York: Penguin Press, 2011.

Duckworth, Angela. *Grit*. New York: Scribner, 2016.

Mattson, Mark P. "Hormesis Defined." *Ageing Research Reviews* 7, no. 1 (2008): 1–7.

The Relational Cross

Bowen, Murray. *Family Therapy in Clinical Practice*. New York: Jason Aronson, 1978.

Porges, Stephen W. *The Polyvagal Theory*. New York: W. W. Norton, 2011.

Conclusion

Cloud, Henry, and John Townsend. *Boundaries*. Grand Rapids, MI: Zondervan, 1992.

Peterson, Eugene H. *Under the Unpredictable Plant*. Grand Rapids, MI: Eerdmans, 1992.

Seligman, Martin E. P. *Flourish*. New York: Free Press, 2011.

Willard, Dallas. *Renovation of the Heart*. Colorado Springs, CO: NavPress, 2002.

Wright, N. T. *Paul and the Faithfulness of God*. Minneapolis: Fortress Press, 2013.

CONTINUE YOUR JOURNEY
Take the SCAL Assessment

Discover your Total Being Fitness profile with our comprehensive 108-question assessment. In just 15 minutes, you'll receive:

- Your personalized archetype (one of 52 unique patterns)
- Detailed analysis of your strengths across all six arenas
- Specific growth recommendations tailored to your profile
- A customized roadmap for your transformation

Visit: saycheeseandlift.com/scal-method-assessment

COMING SOON:
The SCAL Method Implementation Course